Histology of the Striped Bass

David B. Groman

Department of Pathobiology
University of Connecticut
Storrs, Connecticut 06268

American Fisheries Society
Monograph Number 3
ISSN 0362-1715

Bethesda, Maryland
1982

Dedicated to Mary and Walter, whose religious pursuit of the American Dream made it all possible

Publication of this Monograph
was made possible by grants from the
United States Fish and Wildlife Service
Department of the Interior
and the
United States National Marine Fisheries Service
Department of Commerce, National Oceanic and Atmospheric Administration

American Fisheries Society Monographs: ISSN 0362-1715
Library of Congress Catalog Card Number: 82-72542

5410 Grosvenor Lane
Bethesda, Maryland 20814

Contents

Tables

Figures

Plates

Scientific Names of Fish Species Cited in the Text

American eel	*Anguilla rostrata*
Asiatic snakehead	*Channa asiatica*
Black crappie	*Pomoxis nigromaculatus*
Black sea bass	*Centropristis striata*
Bluegill	*Lepomis macrochirus*
Boccacio	*Sebastes paucispinis*
Bowfin	*Amia calva*
Brown trout	*Salmo trutta*
Bullheads	*Ictalurus* spp.
Central stoneroller	*Campostoma anomalum*
Channel catfish	*Ictalurus punctatus*
Cherry (Masu) salmon	*Oncorhynchus masou*
Chinook salmon	*Oncorhynchus tshawytscha*
Common carp	*Cyprinus carpio*
Coral fish	*Chelman rostratus*
Crappies	*Pomoxis* spp.
Cunner	*Tautoglabrus adspersus*
Daces	*Rhinichthys* spp.
European eel	*Anguilla anguilla*
European plaice	*Pleuronectes platessa*
Fathead minnow	*Pimephales promelas*
Gulf menhaden	*Brevoortia patronus*
Guppy	*Poecilia reticulata*
Lancetfishes	Alepisauridae
Largemouth bass	*Micropterus salmoides*
Longjaw mudsucker	*Gillichthys mirabilis*
Mimic shiner	*Notropis volucellus, N. v. buchanani*
Northern pike	*Esox lucius*
Northern searobin	*Prionotus carolinus*
Pimelodid catfishes	*Pimelodus maculatus, P. scrofa*
Rainbow trout	*Salmo gairdneri*
Striped bass	*Morone saxatilis*
Threespine stickleback	*Gasterosteus aculeatus*
Turbot	*Scophthalamus maxima*
White crappie	*Pomoxis annularis*
White sucker	*Catostomus commersoni*
Yellow perch	*Perca flavescens*

Introduction

Several comparative vertebrate histology texts include chapters on fish histology; noteworthy are those by Hoar and Randall (1969), Patt and Patt (1969), Harder (1975), Leake (1975), Ali and Anctil (1976), Welsch and Storch (1976), and Roberts (1978). Although new texts are in preparation, there are available today only two definitive references on fish histology, both concerning members of evolutionarily lower teleost orders. One, published by Anderson and Mitchum in 1974, concerns trout (Salmoniformes) and the other, by Grizzle and Rogers published in 1976, concerns channel catfish (Siluriformes).

Except for descriptions of pathology, only a few papers have been published on striped bass histology. Among these are reports by Merriman (1941) on ovarian tissues, by Faulkner (1952) on the retinas of serranid fishes, by Beitch (1962, 1963) on the urinary system, and by Bryant (1970) and Bryant and Seibel (1970, 1971) on the morphology and ultrastructural development of pronephric and mesonephric tubules. Beitch's work (1962) is especially pertinent as it describes the osmoregulatory histology of anadromous striped bass. He documented changes in the renal excretory histology but did not include comparisons of the other osmoregulatory tissues, such as chloride cells in the gills, integument, digestive mucosa, or urinary bladder.

The striped bass has been both an important food source and sport fish in the United States for more than two centuries. Its life history (Table 1) and commercial importance along the eastern and western coasts of America have been well documented (Pearson 1938; Merriman 1941; Raney 1952; Bigelow and Schroeder 1953; Bradford 1957; Nichols 1966; Barkuloo 1970; Koo 1970). Populations of striped bass are harvested commercially from the St. Lawrence River in Canada to the Gulf of Mexico along the Louisiana coast. This anadromous species also has supported a substantial fishing industry along the Pacific coast since shortly after its introduction there in the latter part of the nineteenth century.

Fishing statistics of the United States Department of Commerce (1972–1973) and of the United Nations (1975) put the average yearly catch of striped bass in the United States at over 2,268 metric tons. These figures represent a 10-fold increase over annual landings recorded in 1934 (Koo 1970). Undoubtedly, the striped bass has come of age as an economically important commercial and sport fish.

In the past 20 years, federal and state governments have begun to establish reproducing populations of striped bass in freshwater environments throughout the United States (Westin and Rogers 1978). Over 21 states presently stock or culture this species to meet the increasing demand for it as a sport fish. Research into histomorphology has not paralleled the demand for the culture of this economically significant species. Recent interest by the United States Fish and Wildlife Service in the diminishing spawning success of the anadromous stocks of striped bass has reinforced the need for this basic research.

From the standpoint of an increasing world demand for an inexpensive and easily obtainable source of dietary protein, aquaculture of striped bass and other marine and anadromous teleosts can help to alleviate protein deficiencies in many parts of the world (Ronsivalli 1976). As for any intensive food-producing enterprise, disease control is of prime importance in maintaining the efficiency of operation and production. This atlas was developed to provide a reference for those concerned with the health maintenance of striped bass propagated under intensive aquaculture conditions. Because it includes discussions and photographs of all major organ systems from normal fish, it also should be useful to those who need to assess abnormal or pathologic changes in field and laboratory specimens.

Acknowledgments

My appreciation is extended to the following people who have made this publication possible through their support, guidance, and assistance.

At the University of Connecticut, Department of Pathobiology: Betty Holzshu and Patricia Timmins for typing several first-draft sections of the manuscript; Robert Pirozok, Head, and Norma Hice, Assistant, of the Histology Laboratory for use of their facilities and for their assistance in the preparation of the tissue specimens and special stains used in this study; David Hill for electron microscopy of selected specimens; Stuart Wyand for serving as an Associate Advisor to the study

Table 1.—*Life-history summary for striped bass.*

Characteristic	Race	Remarks	References[a]
Distribution			
General		*Atlantic coast:* St. Lawrence River, Quebec–New Brunswick to St. Johns River, Florida. *Gulf of Mexico coast:* Escambia River, west Florida to Tchefuncta River, east Louisiana. *Pacific coast:* southern California to British Columbia. *Landlocked:* reservoirs throughout southeastern United States.	2 ,4, 8, 9, 11, 15, 32, 39, 42, 49, 50, 52, 53, 57, 59
Habitat		Tidal rivers, estuaries, bays, open coasts, sandy beaches, rocky areas. *Summer, fall:* coastal areas, shallow to moderately deep saltwater.[b] *Winter:* deeper water at entrances to rivers or bays.[b] *Spring:* brackish estuaries and turbulent freshwater rivers.[b]	As above
Races	A	St. Lawrence River, Quebec–New Brunswick.	4
	B	Hudson River, New York.	26, 31, 38, 43, 60
	C	Upper Chesapeake Bay, Maryland.	26, 27, 35, 38, 43, 60
	D	Lower Chesapeake Bay, James River, Virginia.	26, 27, 35, 38, 43, 60
	E	Albemarle Sound, North Carolina.	27, 44, 59
	F	South Carolina to St. Johns River, Florida (including landlocked populations).	9, 26, 27, 44
	G	Gulf of Mexico, Florida to Louisiana.	4
	H	Pacific coast, southern California to British Columbia.	38, 43
Movements[b]			
Ages 0–1		*Summer, fall, winter:* remain in brackish or saltwater near river months. *Spring:* may run upstream.	28, 46, 47
Ages 2–adult	A	Moderately ranging populations: *summer and fall,* south to New England; *winter,* north to St. Lawrence River area; *spring,* upstream migration to spawn.	4
	B	Moderately ranging populations: *summer and fall,* eastward from Hudson River into Long Island Sound; *winter,* westward to mouth of Hudson River; *spring,* upstream migration to spawn.	1, 3, 4, 6, 8, 31, 45
	C,D	Long-ranging populations: *summer and fall,* northeastward to Long Island and New England; *winter,* southwestward back to Chesapeake Bay area; *spring,* up tributaries of Chesapeake Bay to spawn.	7, 8, 14, 25, 33, 48, 60
		Short-ranging populations: *summer and fall,* into Chesapeake Bay for feeding; *winter,* to deeper holes; *spring,* upstream to spawn.	30, 33, 34, 36, 58
	E,F,G	Limited range: *summer and fall,* into sounds or bays; *winter,* to deeper holes near river mouths; *spring,* upstream to spawn.	7, 14, 60
	H	*Summer,* to brackish or saltwater; *fall, winter, and spring,* upstream until spawning is completed.	7, 37, 40
Diet			
Age 0		Rarely fish, mostly invertebrates: shrimp, copepods, cladocerans, neomysids, insects, decapods, polychaetes, isopods. Begin to eat 4.5–10 days posthatching.	5, 29, 45
Age 1–adult		Voracious predators on a wide variety of fish and invertebrates. *East coast:* anchovies, clupeids, silversides, shiners, shrimp, crabs, lobsters. *West coast:* east-coast groups plus chinook salmon, common carp, crayfish. *Fresh water:* clupeids, crappies, yellow perch, daces, bullheads, leptodorids shrimp, mayfly nymphs.	4, 5, 12, 17, 19, 20, 22, 32, 39, 42, 50, 51, 53, 54
Growth and maturity		*Growth:* first year, about 11 cm; second year, to 22 cm; third year, to 35 cm; fourth year, to 45 cm. *Maturity:* males, most spawning in 2 years; females, 25% spawn after 4 years, 75% after 5 years, 95% after 6 years.	4, 10, 23, 24, 28, 32, 39, 42, 45, 47, 59, 61
Fecundity		200,000 to 700,000 eggs in a 4.5-year-old female.	4, 32, 42
Spawning time		Varied within the period April–July according to temperature and latitude: April–May in North Carolina; May in the Chesapeake Bay area and Hudson River; June in New England; July in the St. Lawrence River area. Spawning females are surrounded by 10–50 small males that fight fiercely with each other. Eggs are 1.10–1.35 mm in diameter when deposited; hatch time (30–74 hours) varies with water temperature (10–22 C).	4, 13, 21

Table 1.—*Continued*

Characteristic	Race	Remarks	References[a]
Place	A,B,C, D,E,F[b]	Brackish estuaries or turbulent areas of freshwater rivers.	4, 11, 21, 23, 32, 39, 42, 49, 52, 55
	F	Landlocked populations: turbulent tributaries.	18, 53
	G	Brackish delta areas primarily, and in freshwater rivers.	16, 41, 56, 62

[a] 1 Alperin (1966a)
2 Alperin (1966b)
3 Austin and Custer (1977)
4 Bigelow and Schroeder (1953)
5 Boynton et al. (1981)
6 Chadwick (1962)
7 Chapoton and Sykes (1961)
8 Clark (1968)
9 Dalberg and Scott (1971)
10 Dey (1981)
11 Dickson (1958)
12 Dovel (1968)
13 Dovel and Edmonds (1971)
14 Dudley et al. (1977)
15 Forester et al. (1972)
16 Hatten (1942)
17 Heubach et al. (1963)
18 Hogue et al. (1977)
19 Hollis (1952)
20 Hughes (1975)
21 Johnson and Koo (1975)
22 Johnson and Calhoun (1952)
23 Kernehan et al. (1981)
24 Koo and Ritchie (1973)
25 Koo and Wilson (1972)
26 Lewis (1957)
27 Lund (1957)
28 Mansueti (1961)
29 Markle and Grant (1970)
30 Massmann and Pacheco (1961)
31 McLaren et al. (1981)
32 Merriman (1941)
33 Moore and Burton (1974)
34 Moore and Burton (1975)
35 Morgan et al. (1973)
36 Nichols and Miller (1967)
37 Orsi (1971)
38 Otto (1975)
39 Pearson (1938)
40 Radovich (1963)
41 Radtke and Turner (1967)
42 Raney (1952)
43 Raney and DeSylva (1953)
44 Raney and Wolcott (1955)
45 Rathjen and Muller (1957)
46 Ritchie and Koo (1973)
47 Robinson (1960)
48 Schaefer (1968)
49 Scruggs (1957)
50 Scruggs and Fuller (1955)
51 Shapovalov (1936)
52 Smith (1907)
53 Stevens (1958)
54 Thomas (1907)
55 Tresselt (1952)
56 Turner (1976)
57 Turner and Chadwick (1972)
58 Vladykov and Wallace (1938)
59 Vladykov and Wallace (1952)
60 Westman and Wallace (1954)
61 Wirtanen and Ray (1971)
62 Woodhull (1947)

[b] Except for landlocked populations.

on which this monograph is based, and for advice concerning the interpretation of the histologic preparations; and Patricia Hopko of the Research Foundation Office who typed most of the manuscript drafts.

At the University of Rhode Island: Deborah Westin and Bruce Roberts, Marine Experiment Station, for the supply of valuable specimens; Richard Wolke, Department of Aquacultural Science and Pathology, who also served as Associate Advisor to this study and who provided valuable guidance on the preparation and interpretation of various specimens; and Peter Belinsky for information on striped bass hematology.

At the University of Idaho, A. J. Chacko helped design the cover.

From the United States Fish and Wildlife Service: Monte Stuckey, Leetown National Laboratory, for photographic guidance and assistance; Elliot Astupenas and his staff, Edenton National Fish Hatchery, for the supply of fish of various ages needed in the study; and Roger Herman, Director, National Fish and Research Development Center, who provided both support for preparation of the many histologic microscope slides, and consultation on their interpretation, and who served as Associate Advisor to this study.

I thank my Major Advisor, C. N. Burke, for suggesting the preparation of this atlas as a Master's Degree project, and for providing unending encouragement, assistance, and professional support during the study and its preparation for publication.

A very special expression of appreciation is due to S. F. Snieszko of the Leetown Laboratory for his generous encouragement and personal involvement in having this work considered for publication.

Methods

Specimens studied were obtained from the University of Rhode Island Marine Experiment Station and the Edenton (North Carolina) National Fish Hatchery. The Rhode Island fish had hatched from eggs obtained from the Moncks Corner State Hatchery in South Carolina. They were reared in tanks where salinity of the water ranged from 28 to 30‰ and the temperature was held at a constant of 22 C year around. The fish were maintained on a diet of squid and commercial feed (Rangen Trout Chow). Specimens provided for this atlas included five 3-week-old larvae, five 3-month-old juveniles, seven age-3 juveniles less than 25 cm long, and two adults older than age 3 and greater than 50 cm long.

The fish obtained from North Carolina were hatched from eggs spawned at the Edenton Hatchery and raised there in ponds where the salinity was less than 5‰ and temperature varied seasonally. Fish were maintained on commercial feed (Silver Cup and Glenco Mills trout diets) in addition to food naturally occurring in the hatchery ponds. Specimens provided for this atlas included three age-3 adults that exceeded 50 cm total length.

Tissue Selection and Fixation

All fish were anesthesized with 0.001–0.003% solutions of Quinaldine (2-methylquinoline, Eastman Kodak). The drug was first dissolved in acetone because of its low solubility in water.

The following organ systems were examined from each specimen: *circulatory and hematopoietic systems* (heart, blood vessels, lymphatic vessels, spleen, head kidney, thymus, blood cells); *digestive system* (buccal cavity, esophagus, stomach, intestines, anus); *extramural organs* (liver, gall bladder, pancreas, gas bladder); *respiratory system* (gills, pseudobranchs); *renal excretory system* (renal corpuscles, renal tubules, urinary bladder); *reproductive system* (testes, ovaries); *integumentary system* (skin, fins, scales); *muscular system* (smooth muscle, skeletal muscle, cardiac muscle); *skeletal system* (acellular bone, spongy bone, mixed bony tissue, chondroid, gill cartilage, hyaline cartilage); *nervous system* (myelencephalon, metencephalon, mesencephalon, diencephalon, telencephalon, spinal cord, peripheral nerves); *sensory structures and organs of special sense* (olfactory organ, eye, inner ear, lateral line, superficial neuromasts, taste buds); and *endocrine system* (interrenal gland, chromaffin tissue, corpuscles of Stannius, pituitary gland, thyroid gland, urophysis, endocrine pancreas, ultimobranchial bodies).

The fixatives used were acetic-formol-sublimate (Bucke 1972), formol-acetic acid-alcohol (Bucke 1972), Bouin's solution (Humason 1972), Zenker's fixative (Humason 1972), Helly's fixative (Humason 1972), 10% neutral buffered formalin (Humason 1972), buffered glutaraldehyde (Humason 1972), Bouin's–Allen's fixative (Gabe 1976), and Serra's fixative, which includes alcohol–formaldehyde–glacial acetic acid in a ratio of 4:2:1. The eyes, gills, digestive mucosa, gall bladder, and nervous tissue, which deterioriate rapidly, were preserved first. The alimentary tract was perfused through both the esophageal and anal openings to insure proper preservation. After fixation, all tissues were rinsed or stored in 70% alcohol or processed directly for histology.

Light Microscopy

With the exception of some liver samples, which were frozen for cryostat sectioning, and gill tissues which were fixed for electron microscopy, all samples were processed, embedded in paraffin, and sectioned at 5–7 μm in compliance with accepted histological procedures (Luna 1967; Humason 1972; Gabe 1976). The cryostat sections of the liver were stained for fat and glycogen deposits with the oil-red-O (ORO) and Best's carmine (BC) techniques, respectively (Humason 1972). The paraffin sections were routinely stained with either a regressive Harris' hematoxylin and eosin (H&E) stain or with a hematoxylin–phloxine–saffron trichrome technique (Luna 1967).

Special stains were used to demonstrate specific histological structures: phosphotungstic acid-hematoxylin (PTAH) (Levene and Feng 1964) for alpha cells in the endocrine pancreas; Gomori's aldehyde fuchsin (AF) (Scott 1952) for beta cells of the endocrine pancreas; Grossman's modification of Mallory's triple stain (GT)[1] for muscle,

[1] This modification of Mallory's triple stain was developed at the University of Minnesota Veterinary School. Copies of the protocol can be obtained through the Head, Histology Laboratory, Department of Pathobiology, University of Connecticut, Storrs, Connecticut 06268.

connective and epithelial tissues; azocarmine and aniline blue (Azan) (Mallory-Heidenhain) (Gabe 1976) for endocrine and neurosecretory cells of the pituitary and urophysis; alcian blue-periodic acid-Schiff technique (ABPAS) (Luna 1967) for mucoid cells of the alimentary tract, skin, semicircular canals, and olfactory mucosa; chrome hematoxylin-phloxine technique (CHP) (Gabe 1976) for pituitary cells; Gridley's reticulum stain (GR) (Luna 1967) for reticular fibers in the liver and hepatopancreas; crystal violet-orange G technique (CVOG) (Gabe 1976) for neurosecretory products in the urophysis and pituitary; aldehyde fuchsin (Halmi) technique (AFLG) (Gabe 1976) for pituitary cells; Giemsa and Wright's blood stains (Humason 1972) for blood cells.

Where possible, identical regions of each organ system were sectioned and stained from the different specimens. When necessary, samples containing bone or cartilage were decalcified according to standard procedures (Luna 1967; Hamason 1972; Gabe 1976) to insure uniform sectioning.

Light photomicroscopy was done with Zeiss equipment. Kodak Panatonic-X film was used for all of the black and white photography, and Kodak Kodachrome II Professional Type A slide film for all color photography.

Electron Microscopy

The tissues for electron microscopy were placed in cold (4 C) fixative containing 4% glutaraldehyde, 0.1 M sodium phosphate, and 0.1 M sucrose, final concentration. Within 1 hour, the initial fixative was replaced to minimize dilution by tissue fluids and the specimens remained in the fresh fixative for a period of not less than 24 hours nor more than 1 week. When the weekly processing of fixed tissues was to begin, the tissues were trimmed to sizes that did not exceed 0.5 mm in any two dimensions. The pieces were then washed in cold sucrose-phosphate buffer, dehydrated through a graded ethanol series, and embedded in epon-araldite. Thick sections (0.5 to 1.0 μm) for light microscopic examination were cut with glass knives with an LKB Ultrotome-3 (Stockholm, Sweden), and subsequently stained with toluidine blue (TB; Humason 1972). Thin sections for electron microscopic examination were similarly cut at approximately 20 to 50 nm and stained with uranyl acetate followed by lead citrate (UALC; Gabe 1976). Specimens were examined with Jeol T_6S and 6C electron microscopes and photographed on Kodak Electron Image Plates.

General Anatomy

The striped bass is a member of the order Perciformes, family Perichthyidae (temperate basses), and is a good example of a higher-order bony fish. Its major organ systems are composed of cellular elements common to all vertebrates: skeletal, smooth, and cardiac muscle; epithelial tissues; cartilage and collagenous connective tissue; neurons; and specialized epithelial secretory cells, to name a few. The striped bass body is supported by an internal skeleton of cartilage and acellular bone that compose the skull, vertebral column, ribs, and fin rays or lepidotrichia (Fig. 1). Some major organs (heart, liver, intestines, gall bladder, trunk kidney, brain, and spinal cord) are easily identifiable in sagittal section (Fig. 2). The prominance of brain and spinal-cord tissue in the juvenile shown in Fig. 2 indicates the relative importance of nervous tissue to the survival and development of young fish.

In the following sections, histological details of the major organs are presented. Figures 1 and 2 are guides to the placement of these organs.

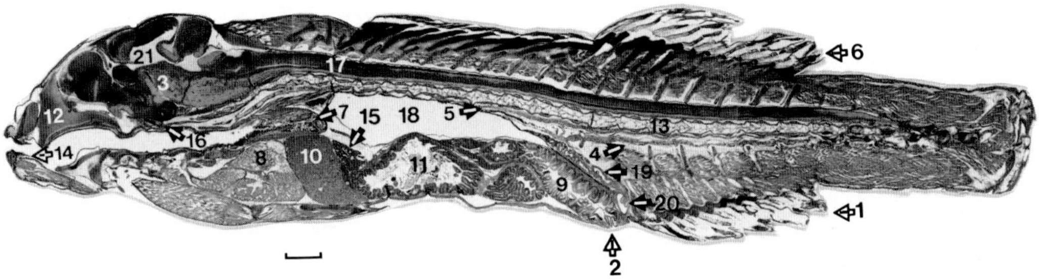

Figure 1. Sagittal section of a 3-month-old striped bass (Bouin's; H&E). Bar = 354 μm.

1 Anal fin
2 Anus
3 Brain
4 Caudal vein
5 Dorsal aorta
6 Dorsal fin
7 Esophagus
8 Heart
9 Rectum
10 Liver
11 Anterior intestine
12 Neurocranium
13 Notochord
14 Oral valve
15 Pancreas
16 Pituitary
17 Spinal cord
18 Gas bladder
19 Trunk kidney
20 Urinary bladder
21 Ventricle of brain

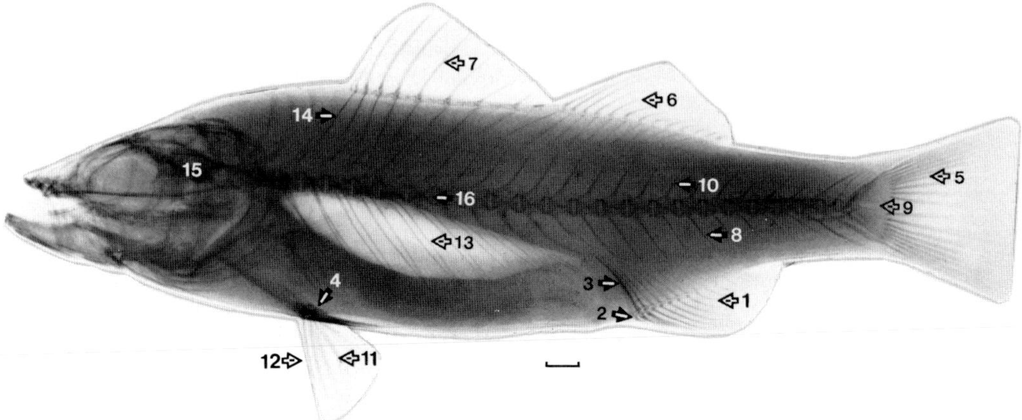

Figure 2. X-ray sagittal view of a juvenille striped bass, 29 cm total length. Bar = 1 cm.

1 Anal fin, lepidotrichia
2 Anal fin, spine
3 Anal pterygiophore
4 Basipterygia
5 Caudal fin, lepidotrichia
6 Dorsal fin, lepidotrichia
7 Dorsal fin, spine
8 Hemal spine
9 Hypural plate
10 Neural spine
11 Pelvic fin, lepidotrichia
12 Pelvic fin, spine
13 Pleural rib
14 Pterygiophore
15 Skull
16 Vertebra

Circulatory and Hematopoietic Systems

The teleost circulatory system, like that of all vertebrates, has two elements: fluid blood tissue and an elaborate vascular component through which the blood moves. The blood comprises liquid plasma and cellular elements (erythrocytes, leukocytes, and thrombocytes). The plasma transports nutrients, essential chemical components, dissolved gasses, metabolic waste products, and chemical buffers (Satchell 1971; Anderson and Mitchum 1974; Harder 1975; Grizzle and Rogers 1976). The cellular elements transport oxygen and provide for both humoral and cell-mediated immunity. The vascular component is composed of the heart, arteries, veins, lymphatic vessels, and sinuses, all of which are lined by endothelium.

Teleosts have a single-pass system for blood flow (Harder 1975). Deoxygenated venous blood is received by the heart and pumped through the gills, reoxygenated, and then distributed to the rest of the body before it returns to the heart. Oxygen concentration and blood pressure vary significantly between arterial and venous blood in such a system (Satchell 1971).

Heart

This specialized muscular enlargement of the blood vessels is responsible for pumping the blood throughout the circulatory system. It is located within the pericardial sac which lies ventral to the buccal cavity and rostral to the liver (Fig. 1). A transverse septum separates the pericardial sac from the peritoneal cavity. As noted above, the blood pumped from the heart must pass through the gill lamellae before moving to the other organs. Consequently, the pressure produced by the heart must be substantial enough to maintain the blood flow to peripheral tissues. Muscular pressure actively aids venous blood in its return to the heart; but blood pressure at the entrance of the sinus venosus of the heart may be negative (Satchell 1971). In such a case, blood is drawn from the hepatic vein into the heart.

The striped bass heart has four compartments: sinus venosus, atrium, ventricle, and bulbus arteriosus (Fig. 3A). These compartments develop from widenings of the embryonic blood vessels or their analogs in the yolk sac of most fish (Harder 1975). Blood enters the sinus venosus via the hepatic (Fig. 3B) and common cardinal veins. It moves through the sinoatrial valve into the atrium and then passes through the atrioventricular valve into the muscular ventricle. Finally, blood is pumped out of the ventricle past the semilunar valves into the bulbus arteriosus and then into the ventral aorta.

The walls of the heart compartments have three tissue layers: epicardium, myocardium, and endocardium (Fig. 3C). The epicardium is continuous with the lining of the pericardial sac. This layer covers the surface of the heart and consists of a pericardial mesothelium supported by connective tissue. Most of the coronary blood vessels, which supply the heart walls, are located in the epicardium. The central myocardium forms the major portion of the walls and is composed of specialized cardiac muscle (refer to section on the Muscular

---

Figure 3. Cardiovascular system of striped bass.

A. Sagittal section of the heart, 3-month-old fish (formalin; H&E). Bar = 81 μm.
B. Hepatic vein between the liver and sinus venosus, 3-month-old fish (formalin; H&E). Bar = 44 μm.
C. Atrial wall (left) and transverse septum (right), 3-year-old juvenile (formol sublimate; H&E). Bar = 44 μm.

1 Atrioventricular valve
2 Atrium
3 Bulbus arteriosus (cordis)
4 Cartilage of the gill arches
5 Endocardium of the atrium
6 Epicardium of the atrium
7 Hepatic vein
8 Liver
9 Myocardium of the atrium
10 Buccal cavity
11 Ostium arteriosum
12 Pharyngeal teeth
13 Proximal value of the bulbus arteriosus
14 Red blood cells
15 Sinoatrial valve
16 Sinus venosus
17 Transverse septum
18 Ultimobranchial body
19 Ventral aorta
20 Ventricle

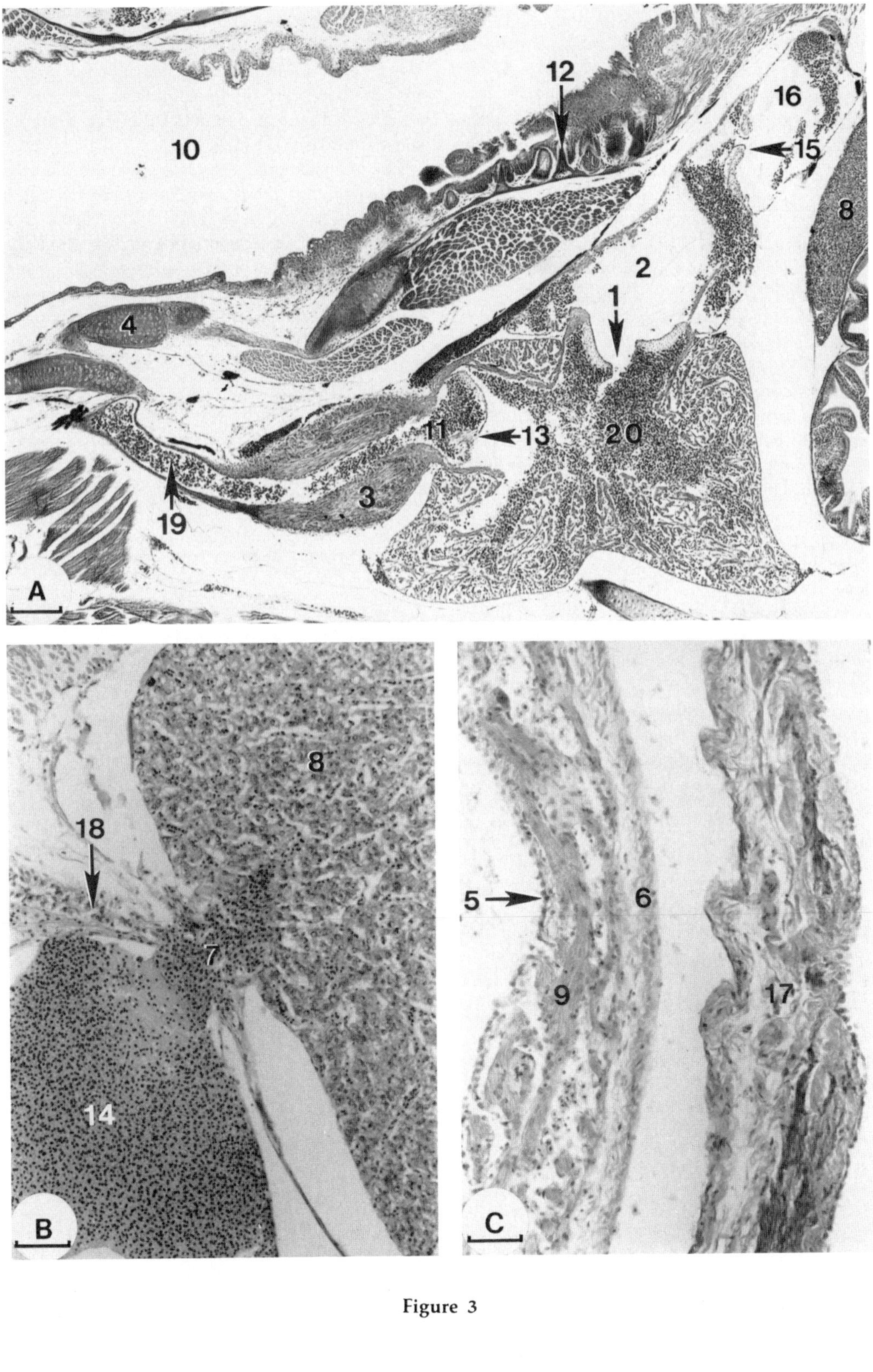

Figure 3

System, page 64). A thin layer of connective tissue separates the myocardium from a thin endocardium. It is the endocardium that forms the lining of the heart and its paired semilunar valves according to Grizzle and Rogers (1976).

In striped bass, the sinus venosus has a thin wall consisting of epicardial and endocardial layers (Fig. 3B). No organized myocardium exists, although a few scattered cardiac muscle fibers are present. This sinus functions as a storage chamber for incoming venous blood. The transverse septum adjoins the sinus venous at its confluence with the hepatic vein (Fig. 3B).

The atrium lies rostral and ventral to the sinus venosus, separated from it by paired sinoatrial valves (Fig 3A). The atrium has a thin epicardium with few coronary blood vessels. The atrial myocardium forms a thin yet distinct layer. Blood can penetrate between the myocardial fibers all the way to the epicardium (Fig. 3C). A thin endocardium lines this chamber and nuclei of its endothelial cells often protrude into the lumen. Macrophages and coarse eosinophilic granular leukocytes are present within the epi- and myocardial layers of the atrium.

The atrioventricular valve is located within the ventral wall of the atrium and opens into the ventricle (Figs. 3A, 4A). The epicardium of the ventricle is thicker than that of the atrium. It has more areolar connective tissue and contains a prominent coronary vascular system (Fig. 4B). The ventricular myocardium is also much thicker than that of the atrium, having both an outer corticalis and an inner spongiosa (Fig. 4B). The densely packed myocardial fibers of the corticalis are oxygenated by capillaries from the coronary vessels. In contrast, the spongiosa is a looser network of anastomosing cardiac muscle bundles enclosed within a thin endocardium. Venous blood, which flows freely between the muscle bundles of the spongiosa, provides oxygen to the muscle fibers. Numerous coarse eosinophilic granular leukocytes occur in the myocardium and epicardium of the ventricle. In addition, aggregates of macrophages and small centers of hematopoiesis are present within the connective tissue of the epicardium in some adult fish (Fig. 4D).

The ventricle opens rostrally, through the posterior semilunar valves, into the bulbus arteriosus (Fig. 4C). The bulbus is composed of elastic connective tissue and smooth muscle fibers (Fig. 4E). It has a thin epicardium and endocardial layer. The myocardium is arranged in dense circular bundles externally and anastomosing lamellar folds internally (Fig. 5A). The bulbus arteriosus narrows rostrally to form the elastic ventral aorta (Fig. 5B). Because of the absence of cardiac muscle in the bulbus, Harder (1975) suggested that it could be considered the first portion of the arterial system in teleosts. The elastic nature of the bulbus arteriosus helps equalize blood-pressure waves from the ventricle, allowing the blood leaving via the ventral aorta to flow more evenly through the delicate capillaries of the gill lamellae.

Blood Vessels

Veins (Fig. 5C–E), arteries (Fig. 5D,E), capillaries (Fig. 5F), and lymph vessels (Fig. 5D) transport fluid in the striped bass. Arteries and veins have an inner tunica intima, a tunica media, and a outer tunica adventitia. The capillaries and smaller lymphatic vessels have only an endothelial layer; larger lymph vessels may have supportive connective tissue (Harder 1975) although none were noted in striped bass.

Veins

Teleost veins are much less rigid than the arteries and often appear collapsed in tissue sections. They contain pocket-shaped, sigmoid, or semilu-

---

Figure 4. Cardiovascular system of a 3-year-old striped bass.

A. Atrioventricular valve of the heart (formol sublimate; H&E). Bar = 222 μm.
B. Coronary blood vessels within the epicardium of the ventricle (formalin; H&E). Bar = 75 μm.
C.. Proximal valve of the bulbus arteriosus (formol sublimate; H&E). Bar = 94 μm.
D. Myocardium of the bulbus arteriosus (formol sublimate; PTAH). Bar = 18 μm.

1 Atrioventricular valve
2 Atrium
3 Bulbus arteriosus
4 Coronary blood vessels
5 Corticalis
6 Endocardial epithelium
7 Epicardium
8 Myoelastic tissue
9 Proximal valve (semilunar valve)
10 Red blood cells
11 Spongiosa
12 Ventricle
13 Ventricular sinus

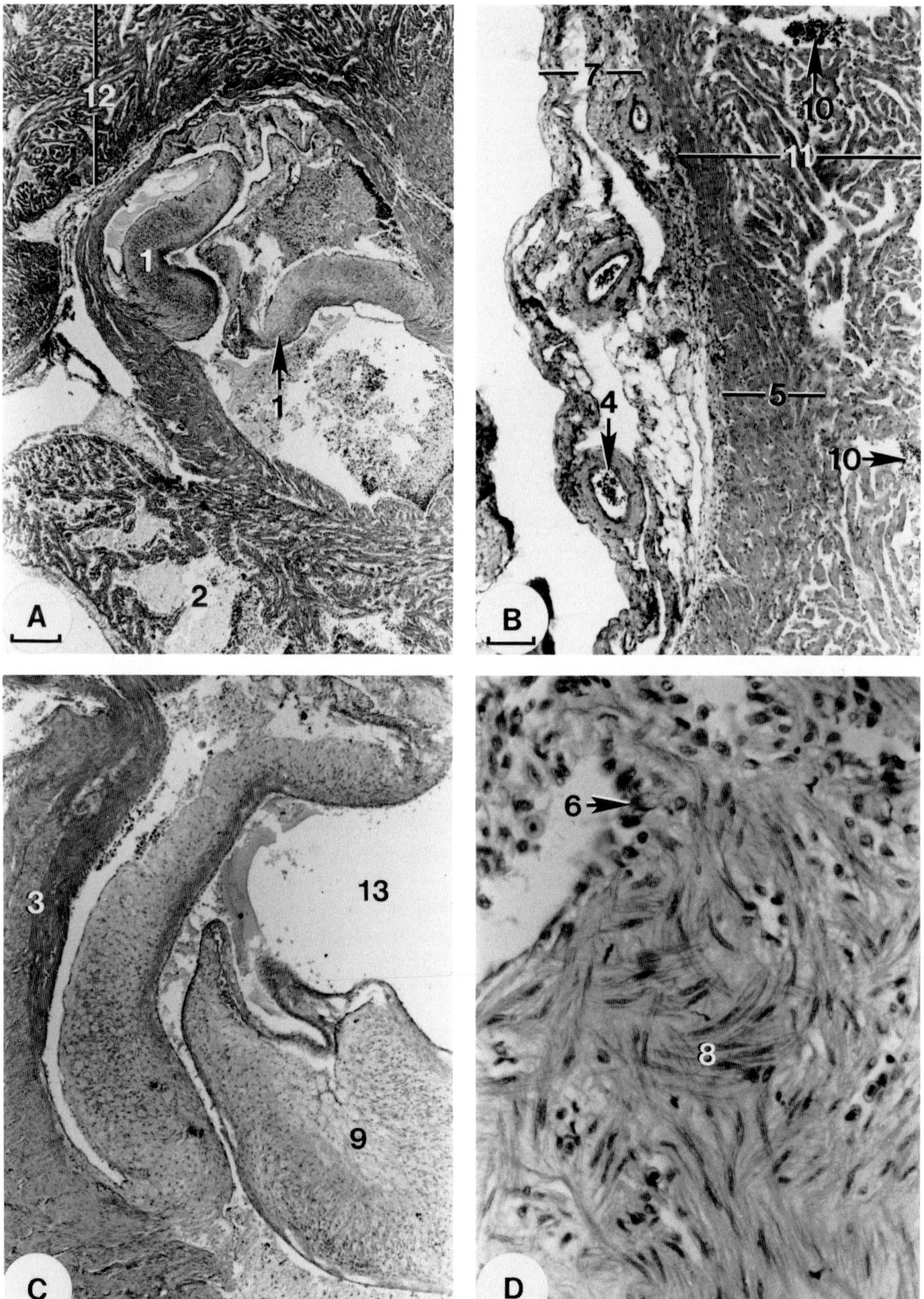

Figure 4

nar valves formed from the endothelium of the tunica intima. These valves generally are paired in veins, as in arteries, and help maintain a consistent flow of blood. Both the tunica intima and tunica media are reduced in the veins and contain less connective tissue and smooth muscle than arteries. The tunica adventitia makes up most of the venous wall and is substantially larger in veins that exit visceral organs and the body wall, as seen, for example, in hepatic portal veins. In some regions of the circulatory system, the veins widen to form blood sinuses such as portions of the posterior cardinal veins of the kidneys (refer to section on Renal Excretory System, page 48) and the jugular veins, which lie dorsal to the ventral aorta (Fig. 5A,B). The veins return deoxygenated blood to the heart and rely on muscular body activity to propel this blood (Satchell 1971).

Arteries

Teleost arteries are lined by a squamous endothelium, which can have nuclei that protrude into the vascular lumen (Fig. 5D,E). This intimal lining occurs throughout all of the vascular organs except the spleen and portions of the liver and head kidney, where the endothelial lining of the sinusoids may be incomplete. An inner elastic membrane and a thin layer of connective tissue are present between the endothelium and the middle layer of the vessel wall (tunica media), which consists of smooth muscle cells that help in the constriction and dilation of the vessel. The tunica media is significantly larger in the arteries than the veins. In some of the larger arteries of the striped bass, it is bordered outside by an external elastic membrane. The tunica adventitia forms the outer wall of the arteries and consists of a connective-tissue fiber lattice with some longitudinal smooth muscle fibers. This connective tissue attaches the blood vessel to surrounding tissue (Harder 1975).

Two types of arteries are found in striped bass: elastic and muscular. The former are best identified by selective staining of the elastic fibers with the para-aldehyde-fuchsin technique (Luna 1967), and, like the ventral aorta and afferent branchial arteries (refer to section on the Respiratory System, page 40), are located closer to the heart. The elastic arteries are able to absorb the higher blood pressure associated with blood pumped directly from the heart to the gills. The muscular arteries contain reduced amounts of elastic fibers (Plate 1A) but more smooth muscle cells within the tunica media. These arteries constitute the bulk of the efferent arteries in the body. Like veins, muscular arteries also contain semilunar valves that develop from the intimal wall and help to prevent back-flushing of blood in the more peripheral arteries (Fig. 5F).

Capillaries

The capillaries comprise the narrowest units of the vascular system (Fig. 6A,B). Their walls consist of only a single layer of endothelial cells reinforced externally by pericytes (Harder 1975). These minute blood vessels are important elements of the circulatory system because they allow the exchange of materials between the blood and other body tissue. Capillary beds also form the connection between the arterial and venous circulation (Grizzle and Rogers 1976).

Striped bass have two elaborate capillary networks or retia mirabilia, one in the ventral wall of the gas bladder and the other comprising the choroid body of the eye (Fig. 6B). These specialized capillary beds permit the concentration and increased exchange of gases from the blood to the gas bladder and retina, respectively. In addition,

Figure 5. Cadiovascular system of a 3-year-old striped bass.

A. Transverse section through the bulbus arteriosus (formalin; H&E). Bar = 120 μm.
B. Transverse section through the ventral aorta (formol sublimate; GT). Bar = 222 μm.
C. Valve of a hepatic portal vein (formalin; HPS). Bar = 23 μm.
D. Blood vessels in dermis near the olfactory bulb (formol sublimate; H&E). Bar = 43 μm.
E. Enlargement from **D** (formalin; H&E). Bar = 23 μm.
F. Mesenteric artery (formalin; H&E). Bar = 63 μm.

1 Areolar connective tissue
2 Bulbus arteriosus
3 Endothelial lining
4 Exocrine pancreatic tissue
5 Fat cells
6 Jugular vein
7 Lymph vessel
8 Muscular artery
9 Olfactory nerve bundle
10 Red blood cells
11 Semilunar valve
12 Tunica adventitia
13 Tunica intima
14 Tunica media
15 Vein
16 Ventral aorta

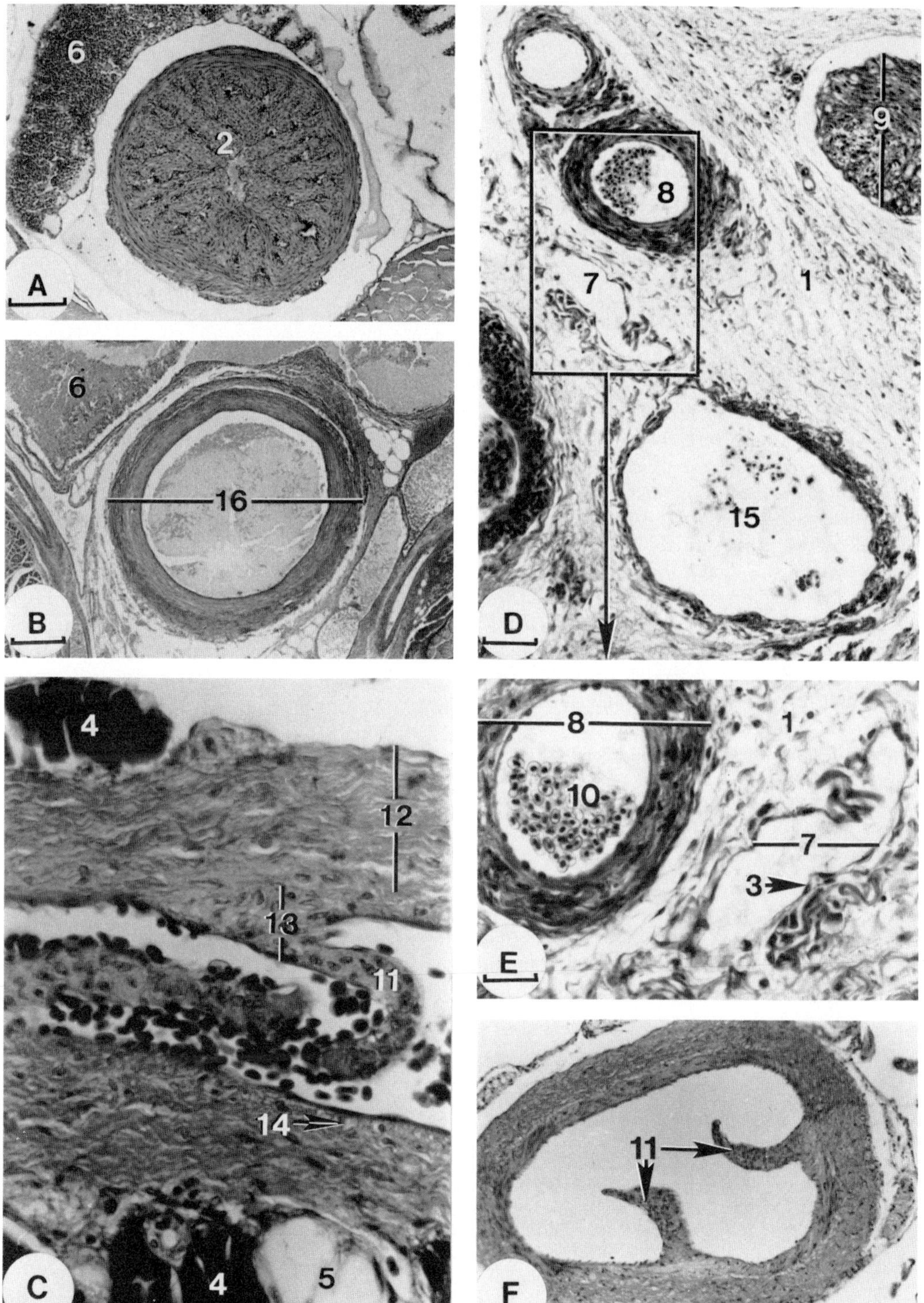

Figure 5

it should be noted that the spleen has lacunae and the liver has sinusoids instead of distinct capillaries. Capillary organizations in the gas bladder (page 38), eye (page 88), spleen (page 16), and liver (page 36) are discussed in greater detail in the respective sections on these structures.

Lymphatic Vessels

The lymphatic system of teleosts, although well developed, has only received slight morphologic and histologic study (Harder 1975). Lymph vessels originate as blind ducts in the submucosa of the alimentary tract, the subcapsular region of the spleen and liver, and beneath the serosa of visceral organs and other tissues. These small lymph vessels unite to form larger ducts that parallel the venous system and eventually empty into it. Harder (1975) stated that the walls of smaller lymph ducts consist of only a single endothelial layer without supporting pericytes or connective tissue, whereas the larger vessels contain some external connective tissue and scattered smooth muscle cells. In this study, the lymphatic system of the striped bass was not examined in detail, but vessels, in conjunction with dermal arteries and veins (Fig. 5D,E), that structurally resembled those described above, were observed. The lymphatic system transports lymph fluid and leukocytes away from the tissues and eventually deposits them into the venous circulation proximal to the sinus venosus.

Hematopoietic Tissues

Hematopoiesis in teleosts may occur along the reticuloendothelial stroma of the vascular system and its associated organs (heart, thymus, spleen, kidney, and liver) or within other body tissues such as the submucosa of the intestines (Harder 1975; Grizzle and Rogers 1976). In the striped bass, germinal centers of hemoblasts were most numerous within the head kidney and spleen of adult and juvenille fish (Fig. 7A). However, foci were also evident within the liver, trunk kidney (Fig. 20C), epicardium of the heart (adult fish primarily), and thymus.

Thymus

The thymus has been considered an endocrine organ, a hematopoietic organ, and an organ of prime importance in the immune system (Tamura and Honma 1977). Functions attributed to it include production of thymosin to stimulate the immune response, development of thymocytes into hemoblasts, and maturation of lymphocytes.

The striped bass thymus is histologically more prominent in juvenile fish where its size is proportionately greater than at any other stage of growth. It is located between the epithelium and the dermis at the superior edge of the gill cover in the opercular cavity (Harder 1975) (Fig. 6C,D). This hematopoietic organ is enclosed by a thin connective tissue capsule that forms a lacuna subdivided by a fine reticular stroma. Thymocytes, which appear as small lymphocytes, constitute the predominant cell type (Plate 1B). In addition, larger lymphocytes, macrophages (Plate 1C), and some coarse eosinophilic granular leukocytes are present (Plate 1D). The density of these cellular components is greater in the peripheral region. Thus, the striped bass thymus is loosely divided into a cortex and medulla (Fig. 6D), similar to that described for the channel catfish by Grizzle and Rogers (1976) (Fig. 6D).

The thymus is most important during immunogenesis in young fish. Again, this is best exemplified by its relatively large size in young-of-the-year fish. As the striped bass matures, the thymus does not grow at a rate proportional to the

---

Figure 6. Circulatory and hematopoietic systems of striped bass.

- **A.** Dermal capillary, 3-year-old fish (formol sublimate; H&E). Bar = 49 μm.
- **B.** Rete mirabile of the eye, 3-year-old fish (formalin; HPS). Bar = 18 μm.
- **C.** Parasagittal section of buccal cavity through the thymus, 3-month-old fish. (formalin; H&E). Bar = 261 μm.
- **D.** Transverse section of the thymus, 3-month-old fish (formalin; H&E). Bar = 82 μm.
- **E.** Macrophage aggregation in the ventricular epicardium of the heart, 3-year-old fish (formalin; H&E). Bar = 27 μm.

1 Aerolar connective tissue
2 Buccal cavity
3 Cartilage of gill arch
4 Corticalis
5 Endothelium
6 Epicardium
7 Gill lamellae
8 Macrophages
9 Mucosal epithelium
10 Neurocranium
11 Pseudobranch
12 Red blood cells
13 Retina of eye
14 Semicircular canals
15 Skeletal muscle bundles
16 Thymic cortex
17 Thymic medulla
18 Thymus

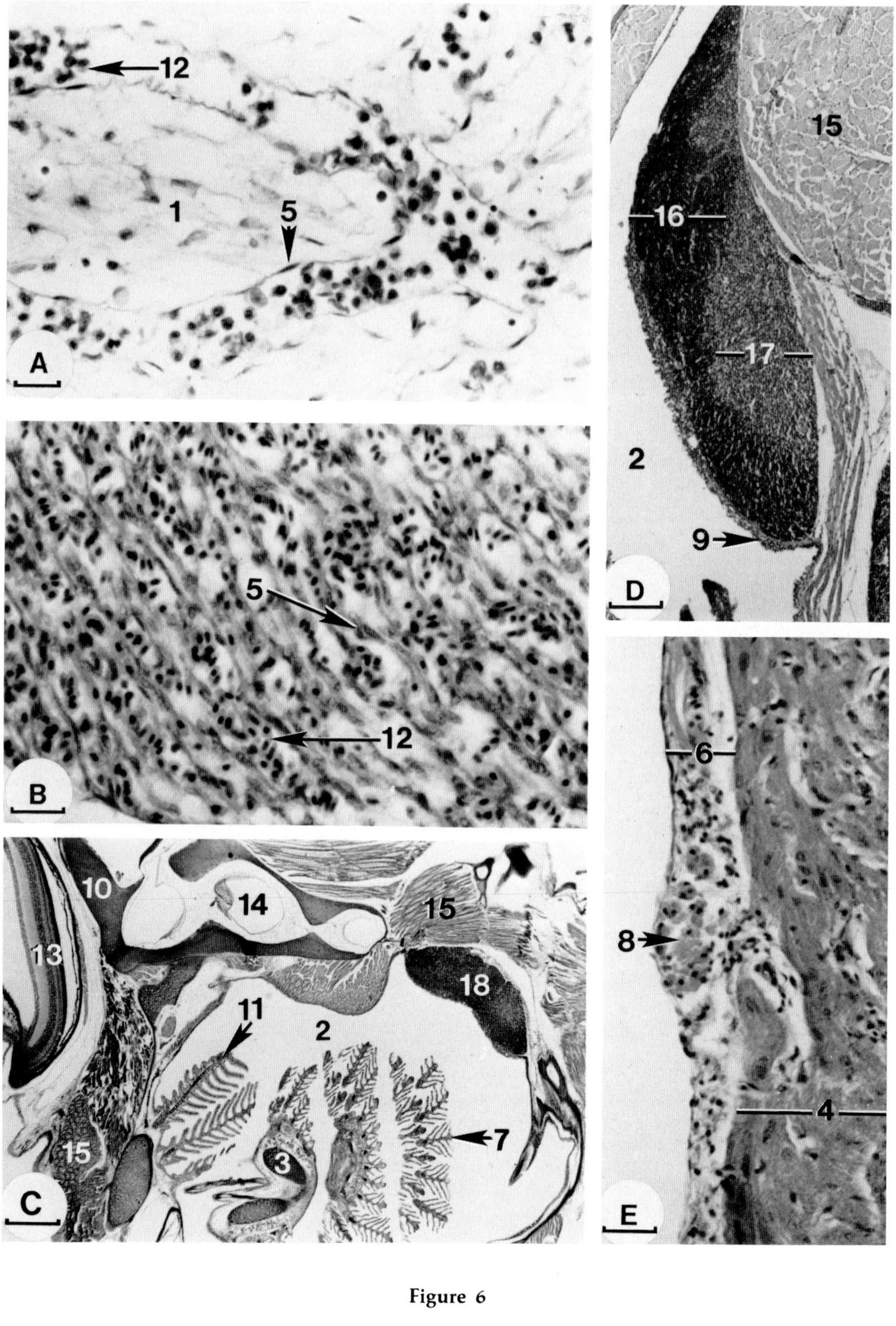

Figure 6

rest of the body. Rather, only the connective tissue of the vascular walls increases, Hassall's corpuscles appear, cyst formation of epitheloid cells occurs, and, with the advent of spawning, the organ may regress as it does with gobiid fishes (Tamura and Homna 1977).

The coarse eosinophilic granular leukocytes described above are most often found in the submucosa of the alimentary tract, the mesenteric fat, pancreatic connective tissue, gill lamellae, the wall of the heart, below epithelial layers, and along connective tissue septa of soft tissues of the striped bass. In contrast to a report that such cells could be found in blood and spleen of yellow perch (Cotton 1951), none were observed in similar fixed tissues of the striped bass. This could be due to fixation and the fragile nature of these cells. The description by Lester and Daniels (1976) of tissue eosinophils of the white sucker closely resembles the coarse eosinophilic granular leukocytes found in striped bass; oval to pleomorphic cells, each with a compact, sometimes indented, and always eccentrically placed nucleus (Plate 1D). Their cytoplasm contains large round to oval eosinophilic granules when stained by common blood and tissue stains.

These cells long have been controversial because little is known about their function. Roberts (1978) considered them to be separate from blood-borne eosinophils and Barber and Westerman (1978) found that the cytoplasmic granules could be stained by the periodic acid–Schiff (PAS) method in many species of fish. Lester and Daniels (1976) also suggested that they were identical to the finely reticular cell of the blood in the white sucker. It was their contention that these peroxidase-negative cells were more closely related to human neutrophils than human eosinophils. However, blood granulocytes stain peroxidase-positive in the striped bass, indicating that the coarse eosinophilic granular leukocytes are unrelated to them. Ezeasor and Stokoe (1980) examined similar cells from the gut of rainbow trout. They determined that the granules contain phospholipid, acid mucopolysaccharide, and the activities of alkaline phosphatase, acid phosphatase, arylsulphatase, and 5-nucleotidase. Work by Ellis et al. (1981) suggests that these cells of trout degranulate like mammalian mast cells and may contain histamine.

Spleen

The spleen is an important lympho-myeloid organ in fish. This elongated triangularly shaped organ is located along the hepatic portal veins that follow the dorsal mesentery between the gall bladder and the liver (Fig. 7A). It is contained within a thin fibrous connective tissue capsule, which is covered by a single layer of mesothelial cells. The spleen is penetrated by the splenic artery, vein, parasympathetic nerve bundles, and, at the entrance of its major blood vessels, by pancreatic exocrine acini. Capillary branches of the central artey and vein, termed ellipsoids, and a spongy cellular reticulum, comprise the stroma of the teleost spleen (Yoffey 1929). Trabeculae are absent.

Bach et al. (1978) noted that the splenic pulp of the channel catfish consists of a loosely arranged meshwork of reticulum and reticular cells that forms channels or lacunae through which blood percolates. In striped bass, the splenic ellipsoids are scattered within the reticular stroma and most of the lympho-myeloid tissue (white pulp) simply surrounds them (Fig. 7B). This myeloid element primarily consists of hemoblasts, lymphocytes, and macrophages (Plate 1E). The remainder of the white pulp is located within rarely occurring germinal foci or around scattered melano-macrophage centers. The red pulp, composed of mature erythrocytes, some erythroblasts, macrophages, and reticular cells that phagocytize obsolete erythrocytes (Plate 1E), fills the rest of the lacunar space (Fig. 7B). These latter two cell types serve in the major function of the spleen, which is to break

---

Figure 7. Spleen and head kidney of a 3-year-old striped bass.

A. Transverse section of the spleen. (formalin; H&E). Bar = 258 μm.
B. Central blood vessels of the spleen (formalin; H&E). Bar = 87 μm.
C. Hematopoietic head kidney tissue (Bouin's; H&E). Bar = 289 μm.
D. Melano-macrophage center in the head kidney (formalin; H&E). Bar = 19 μm.

1. Arterial branches (elipsoids)
2. Splenic arteries
3. Splenic vein
4. Lymphomyeloid and hematopoietic tissue
5. Macrophages
6. Melanin deposits
7. Melano-macrophage center
8. Peripheral nerve
9. Red pulp
10. White pulp

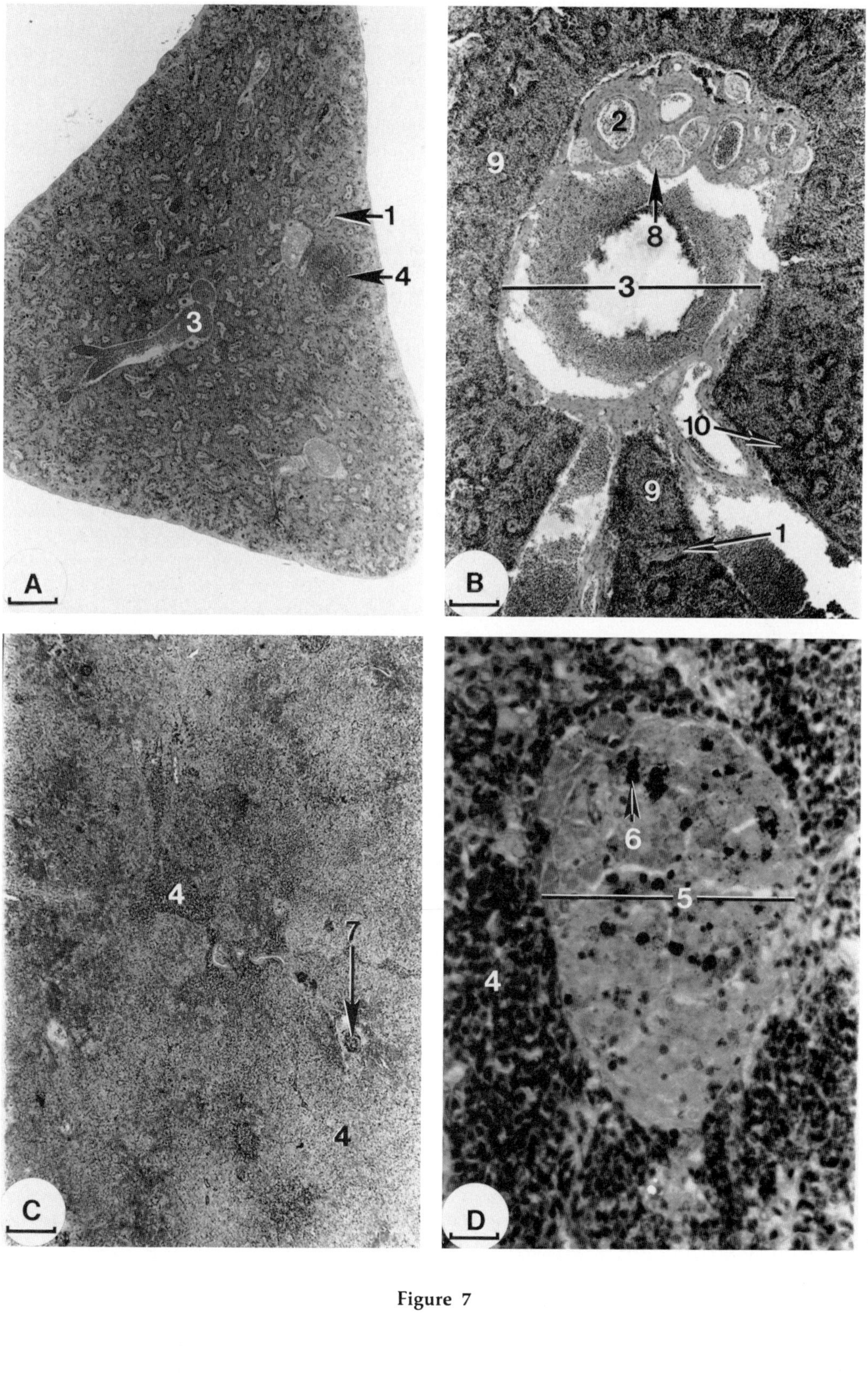

Figure 7

down old erythrocytes and recycle the iron (Agius 1979). In accordance with the observations of Ferguson (1976) for the turbot, fewer hemoblasts and smaller melanin macrophage centers occur in the spleen than in the head kidney of striped bass.

Head Kidney

In striped bass, the head kidney is the rostral continuation of the trunk kidney and contains extensive hematopoietic or lympho-myeloid tissue but few renal tubules (Fig. 7C). This organ is bilobed, covers the entire pharynx, and is fused to the trunk kidney at the fifth intervertebral segment (Beitch 1962). Only the caudal portion of each lobe is ventrally enclosed by a mesothelial layer. Spinal ganglion bundles and the anterior cardinal veins run through the ventral aspect of the head kidney lobes. Branches of these veins directly connect this organ to the circulatory system. In addition, the cortical portion of the right posterior cardinal vein enters the right lobe of the head kidney before joining the common cardinal vein (see Endocrine System, page 94).

Four primary blood cell types make up the hematopoietic element: lymphocytes, hemoblasts, erythroblasts (reticulocytes), and macrophages (Plate 1F). Hemoblasts are predominant within the parenchyma. These omnipresent blood-cell precursors are thought to have the ability to develop into erythroid and myeloid cells (Harder 1975). They are the largest blood cells found in the adult striped bass and have an average size of 10.2 μm. Belinski (Peter Belinski, University of Rhode Island, unpublished data, 1977) noted that they are equal in size to monocytes in juvenile fish. They have a rounded, often eccentrically situated, nucleus that contains loosely arranged chromatin. The cytoplasm stains deeply basophilic and often contains clear vacuoles suggesting a role as a monocyte precursor. The erythroblasts appear in several stages of maturity. These stages (small lymphoid hemoblasts, basophilic erythroblasts, polychromatophilic erythroblasts, acidophilic erythroblasts, and reticulocytes), as described for the Asiatic snakehead by Mahajan and Dheer (1980), are not easily identifiable in striped bass head kidney. The melanin-containing macrophages that occur in the head kidney have condensed, eccentrically placed nuclei, and a vaculated cytoplasm that contains yellow-brick phagocytized debris (lipofucin and melanin), as reported by Agius (1980) for numerous species of fish. In the striped bass these cells stain PAS-positive. This finding is in agreement with those of Roberts (1975) and Agius (1980), both of whom reported on the significance of melano-macrophage centers in the inflammatory response of teleosts. Similar results were obtained by Tokumaru and Ferri (1970) for two species of pimelodid catfishes and common carp, whereas Oguri (1976) stated that these cells in rainbow trout were negative by the PAS method. Pigment-containing macrophages also are found in the spleen but not in the circulation of the striped bass. Splenic melano-macrophages contain some ferric iron pigments when stained by the Perl's Prussian blue method (Gabe 1976), in contrast to those in the head kidney. This finding is in agreement with that of Agius (1979) for 14 species of clinically normal teleost fish.

In striped bass, the melano-macrophages of both the head kidney and the spleen are arranged in centers similar to those described by Agius (1980). These centers are most numerous in the head kidney (Fig. 7C,D) where they are enclosed in a fine argyrophilic capsule and located close to venous branches. Lymphocytes often are located around such centers, suggesting their possible immunologic role in antigen processing (Fig. 7D). Roberts (1975) and Agius (1980) theorized that melano-macrophage aggregates represent primitive analogues to avian or mammalian germinal centers. Aside from this theorized immunologic function, the head kidney serves as a center for blood-cell differentiation of both erythrocytes and leukocytes. In addition, both interrenal and chromaffin tissue is located along the walls of the posterior cardinal veins in this organ (see Endocrine Sytem, page 94).

Blood Cells

Although blood tissue has both a fluid noncellular component and a cellular component, only the histology of blood cells in striped bass was evaluated in this study.The following cell types were noted in the peripheral blood: erythrocytes; reticulocytes; small and large lymphocytes; granulocytes; thrombocytes; and monocytes or macrophages (Plates 1, 2). As noted above, blood cells specific to the thymus (thymocytes), spleen, and head kidney (macrophages and hemoblasts), and other tissue (coarse eosinophilic granular leukocytes) were readily identificable by light microscopy. Cytochemistry and autoradiography, however, were not employed to differentiate the stages of hemoblast development or for the localization of pharmacodynamic tissue granulocytes, such as mast cells.

Erythrocytes

Erythrocytes or red blood cells (Plates 1, 2) are oval in shape and have a round to oval central nucleus with densely packed chromatin. They are the most abundant cell type found in the peripheral blood and function in respiration by transporting oxygen to and carbon dioxide from body tissues (Satchell 1971). According to Belinski (unpublished 1977), they average 8.99 × 5 μm in size for the juvenile striped bass and 11.6 × 6.9 μm in adult fish. Erythrocyte counts ranged from 2.19 × 10^6 cells/ml in juvenile striped bass (Belinski unpublished, 1977) to 5.63 × 10^6 cells/ml in adults (Westin and Rogers 1978).

Reticulocytes

Reticulocytes occur primarily in the spleen and head kidney (Plate 1E,F), but may also be found in peripheral blood (Plate 2A). They contain a large, irregularly shaped, central nucleus of loose chromatin that is surrounded by a light blue-gray cytoplasm when stained by either Giemsa or Wright's blood stains. Maturing reticulocytes have varying degrees of cytoplasm and nuclear condensation and can be distinguished from erythrocytes by their larger size and light blue-gray cytoplasm. Reticulocytes probably develop from omnipresent hemoblasts of the head kidney and spleen (Mahajan and Dheer 1980).

Lymphocytes

Lymphoctyes are agranular leukocytes that occur either as small (5 μm) or large (7 μm) forms in adult striped bass (Plate 2B) and are believed to originate from thymocytes or hemoblasts of the head kidney of teleosts (Harder 1975). According to Belinski (unpublished 1977), they comprise 60% of the total leukocytes in juvenile fish and measure 5.22 μm and 8.05 μm. A nucleus of dense chromatin occupies 80–90% of the cell volume and is surrounded by a basophilic cytoplasm that can appear vacuolated. Pseudopodia, indented nuclei, and irregular cytoplasmic morphology are seen commonly in the larger lymphocytes (Plate 2B). These immunologic cells frequently are found migrating through epithelial and connective tissues (Figs. 13D, 20C) and function in humoral and cellular immunity (Anderson 1974).

Granulocytes

Granulocytes similar to mammalian neutrophils are the largest leukocytes present in the peripheral blood of adult striped bass (Plate 2A). They have small blue-gray cytoplasmic granules and an indented nucleus. No polymorphonuclear granulocytes, basophils, or eosinophils, however, were observed in the blood. Belinski (unpublished 1977) reported that granulocytes make up approximately 28.5% of the leukocytes and measure about 8.29 μm in the juvenile striped bass; however, the average size in adult fish is 9.6 μm. In addition, granulocytes are present within germinal centers that occur along the interductal reticuloendothelium of the truck kidney as well as other hematopoietic tissues. The true function of teleost granulocytes has yet to be established. Roberts (1978) suggested some role in the inflammatory response but indicated that no definitive evidence of phagocytic activity exists.

Thrombocytes

Thrombocytes are the second most common type of blood cell found in striped bass. These nucleated monocytes possess very little cytoplasm and can appear elongated, spiked, or rounded (Plate 2B,C). Their nuclei may be oval, rounded, elongated, or bilobed, depending on the type and stage of thrombocyte development (Harder 1975). Grizzle and Rogers (1976) suggested that the transformation of elongated forms to rounded forms is involved in the clotting proces. Belinski (unpublished 1977) listed the size of elongated thrombocytes in juvenile striped bass as 6.93 × 3.1 μm. The rounded thrombocytes of adult fish average 4.0 μm, smaller than the lymphocytes for which they are often mistaken. Thrombocytes are believed to function in blood clotting by aiding in the conversion of prothrombin to thrombin. Grizzle and Rogers (1976) suggested that they may develop from immature lymphocytes.

Monocytes

Monocytes or circulating macrophages are the second largest leukocyte found in striped bass blood. They measure 8.2 μm in adults and 12.14 μm in juvenile fish (Belinski unpublished 1977). Monocytes have a large irregularly shaped eosinophilic nucleus and a highly vacuolated basophilic cytoplasm (Plate 2D). Harder (1975) thought circulating monocytes were large hemoblasts that are differentiating into macrophages. Roberts (1978) suggested that monocytes are partially differentiated end cells that would develop into mature phagocytes. The specific function of the teleost monocytes, however, still remains a controversy.

Belinski (unpublished 1977) reported a mean leukocyte count of 17.6 × 10^3 cells/ml in juvenile striped bass and the average hematocrit at 29.2%.

Engel and Davis (1964), Courtois (1976), and Westin (1978) demonstrated higher hematocrits for adults: 38.7%, 46.0%, and 47.9%, respectively. These results indicate that packed cell volumes vary considerably between adult and juvenile fish and may be a function of age, diet, sexual maturity, environmental stress, and disease state (Courtois 1976). Harder (1975) also noted that hematocrit values for most teleosts are comparatively low (20–35%) and that they vary considerably depending upon the physiologic condition of the fish. Grizzle and Rogers (1976) stated that the hematocrits for channel catfish varied greatly among adult fish (30–50%) and young of the year (22–35%). They suggested nutritional factors and age as other reasons for this inconsistency.

Digestive System and Extramural Organs

The digestive system is one of the most-studied aspects of fish histology. Noteworthy are works on chinook salmon (Green 1912), black sea bass and sea robin (Blake 1930, 1936), central stoneroller (Rogick 1931), common carp (Curry 1939), bottom feeders and plankton feeders (A1-Hussaini 1946, 1947), rainbow trout (Weinreb and Bilstad 1955), guppy and threespine stickleback (Hale 1965), northern pike (Bucke 1971), cunner (Chao 1973), alepisauroid fishes (Wassersug and Johnson 1976), American eel (Thurmond 1979), and channel catfish (Sis et al. 1979). In addition, a teleost anatomy text by Harder (1975), two histological texts—one on trout by Anderson and Mitchum (1974), the other on channel catfish by Grizzle and Rogers (1976)—and a review article by Fänge and Grove (1979), address the histology of the digestive system in detail.

Striped bass are piscivorous. Bigelow and Schroeder (1953), Goodson (1964), Trent and Hassler (1966), Schaefer (1970), and Manooch (1973) found that the diets of fish 2 years of age and older included smaller soft-rayed fish (clupeids and anchovies) in addition to invetebrates (amphipods, shrimp, mysids) (Table 1). The striped bass alimentary canal reflects this carnivory: large mouth, buccal cavity, and pharynx, short expandable esophagus; large stomach; and relatively short intestinal section.

The teleost digestive system has two functional units: an alimentary tract that serves as a compartment for the assimilation of food; and the extramural organs that function in metabolic processing of the organic and inorganic substances contained within the alimentary tract.

Alimentary Canal

The alimentary canal of the striped bass has five distinct regions: mouth and buccal cavity; pharynx; esophagus; stomach; and intestines. The large buccal cavity and pharynx contain teeth and gill rakers. Woolcott (1957) described the toothed bones of the neurocranium, dentary, premaxillary, vomer, palantine, and lateral tooth bones of the striped bass tongue. In addition, the tongue has teeth at its anterior tip and centrally along the basihyal. Pharyngeal tooth pads commonly are found on the lower and upper pharyngeals, basibranchials, and hypobranchials. All of the teeth in the buccal cavity and pharynx are conical, curve caudally, and protrude slightly above the epithelium. Fink (1981) classified tooth attachment on both the jaw bones and pharyngeal bones of striped bass as Type 2. This type of tooth is not fully ankylosed to the underlying bone, but has a small area of unmineralized collagen at its base. The gill rakers are biserial and dimorphic; they are of the monacanth type in Harder's (1975) classification scheme. The first of the four gill arches bears long, spine-shaped gill rakers whereas the other three have compressed knobs (see Respiratory System, page 42) and all of them have teeth along their mucosal surfaces. The gill rakers form a screen that channels food particles toward the esophagus and protects the gill filaments.

The foregut begins with a short esophagus having thick longitudinal folds and ends with the stomach; there is no grossly discernible anatomical border between the two. The Y-shaped stomach (Harder 1975) is divided into three regions: corpus ventriculi anteriorly; pars pylorica posteriorly; and a gastric cecum or blind sac originating from the greater curvature of the transitional zone between the corpus ventriculi and pars pylorica. The pars pylorica exits the corpus ventriculi ventrally before it terminates as a narrow, highly muscular valve, the pyloric sphincter.

The anterior intestine originates just posterior to the pyloric sphincter, narrowing at the intestinal valve that demarcates it from the rectum. This valve consists of a circular connective tissue flap that extends caudally into the lumen. The diameter of the anterior intestine is wider, and its mucosa more folded, than those of the rectum. In addition, the anterior intestine contains five to seven pyloric ceca that originate just caudal to the pyloric sphincter. These appendages form conical blind sacs that curve dorsally from their point of origin back along the pars pylorica, to which they may be attached by mesenteries.

The alimentary tract is terminated at the anus, which is one of three external openings on the caudoventral surface of the striped bass just anterior to the anal fin; from anterior to posterior these openings are anus, genital pore, and urinary pore.

Mouth, Buccal Cavity, and Pharynx

The mucosa of the mouth, buccal cavity, and pharynx is composed of statified squamous epithelium, which ranges in thickness from seven to nine cells in areas of the pharyngeal pad to three to four cells along the dorsorostral roof of the buccal cavity (Fig. 8A–D). Type-A goblet cells (page 32) are present in the distal epithelium (Plate 2E) and, except in areas of active secretion, they are covered by a layer of squamous epithelium. In histologic section, lymphocytes are present just above the basal layer of mucosal epithelium throughout the buccal cavity and pharynx.

Taste buds occur primarily in the premaxillary epithelium, on the surface of the tongue, and at the distal end of the epithelial folds in the pharynx, in accordance with the observations of Walker et al. (1981) for the fathead minnow. These sensory structures can be distinguished by their bulb-shaped cutis-papilla, capillary loop, myelinated nerve elements, and concentrically arranged sensory epithelium (see Sensory Structures, page 82). Chromatophores often occur in the mucosa surrounding the taste buds (Fig. 8D).

A thin lamina propria underlies the oral mucosa. The submucosa is composed of loose connective tissue except in sections of the dorsorostral oral cavity where it is dense and lacks the vascularization and cell diversity (lymphocytes, blood cells, coarse eosinophilic granular leukocytes, fat cells, fibrocytes) found in loose connective tissue. Longitudinally arranged, striated muscle bundles are present in the submucosa of the pharynx. They originate dorsal to the pharyngeal pad and are continuous with those of the rostral esophageal muscularis.

The partially ankylosed teeth of the buccal cavity and pharynx are composed of a thin acellular enameloid covering and an inner layer of osteodentine; they contain a central pulp cavity (Fig. 8C,E,F) (Patt and Patt 1969). Teleost teeth are part of the cranial dermal skeleton and function in the acquisition of food. According to Fink (1981), the acrodont teeth of the striped bass are attached to underlying dermal bone by acellular root cement and collagen (page 21). Mature teeth have a pulp cavity that contains nerve fibers, connective tissue, and blood vessels, and that is lined by a layer of stellate odontoblasts (scleroblasts) (Cheprakova 1958). In developing teeth, the osteodentine is secreted from the odontoblasts. Similarly, the enameloid covering is produced by two layers of cuboidal ameloblasts, which surround newly deposited osteodentine (Fig. 8E,F). All developing teeth originate within the submucosa tissues of the buccopharyngeal cavity before protruding through the mucosal epithelium as mature teeth.

The stratified squamous epithelium of the tongue is four to seven cells thick (Fig. 8D) and contains taste buds, Type-A goblet cells, and teeth. This mucosa is supported by a dense lamina propria that encircles a central core of loose areolar connective tissue and hyalinized cartilaginous tis-

---

Figure 8. Anterior digestive system of striped bass.

- **A.** Sagittal section of the mouth and the buccal cavity, 3-month-old fish (formalin; H&E). Bar = 64 μm.
- **B.** Transverse section of the buccal cavity, 3-month-old fish (formalin; H&E). Bar = 155 μm.
- **C.** Transverse section of the upper jaw and the premaxillary bone, 3-year-old fish (formalin; HPS). Bar = 244 μm.
- **D.** Rostral end of the tongue, 3-year-old fish (formalin; HPS). Bar = 58 μm.
- **E.** Sagittal section of a developing acrodont tooth, 3-year-old fish (formol sublimate; HPS). Bar = 48 μm.
- **F.** Transverse section of a developing acrodont tooth, 3-year-old fish; the space between the predentine and the ameloblasts is a fixation artifact (formol sublimate; H&E). Bar = 11 μm.

1 Acrodont tooth
2 Ameloblasts
3 Areolar connective tissue
4 Capillaries
5 Cartilage of the gill arches
6 Chondroid
7 Dentary bone
8 Dermis
9 Enamel organ
10 Epidermis
11 Fibrous enamel (enameloid)
12 Jugular veins
13 Melanocytes
14 Musculus adductor, pars hyomandibular
15 Musculus geniohyoideus (geniohyoid muscle)
16 Neurocranium
17 Odontoblasts
18 Oral mucosa
19 Oral papillae
20 Oral valves
21 Outer enamel epithelium
22 Predentine
23 Premaxillary bone
24 Scleroblasts (pulp cells)
25 Spongy bone
26 Ventral aorta

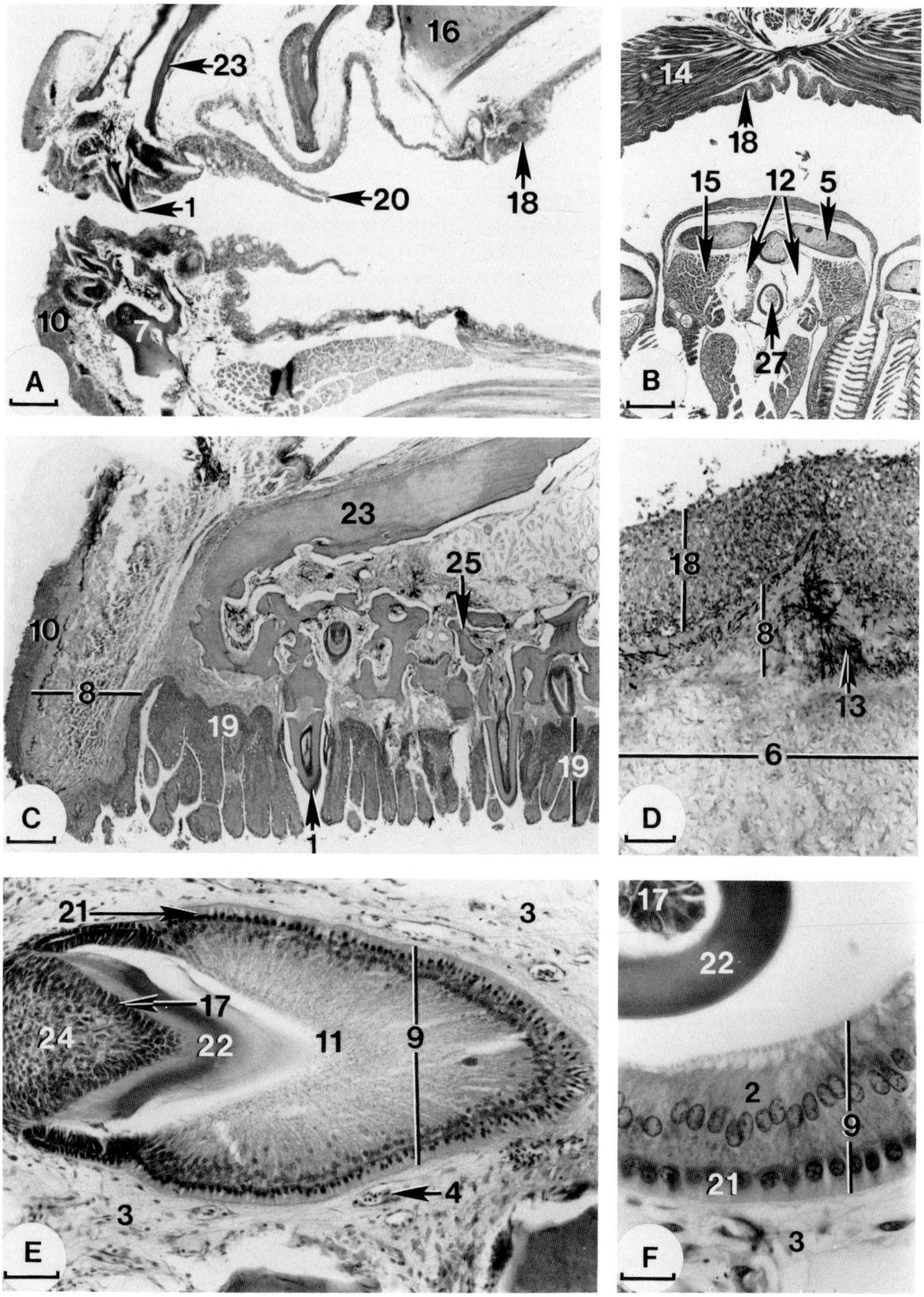

A
23
16
1
20
18
10
7
B
14
18
15
12
5
27
C
23
25
10
8
19
19
1
D
18
8
13
6
E
21
3
17
24
22
11
9
4
3
F
17
22
2
9
21
3

Figure 8

sue elements. No distinct cranial bones or striated muscle elements are present in the tongue anterior to the basihyal bone.

Foregut: Esophagus

The short esophagus begins in the pharynx and continues to the corpus ventriculi of the stomach. The primary, secondary, and tertiary longitudinal folds of its inner mucosal surface expand to aid in swallowing (Fig. 9A–E). Four concentric layers—tunica mucosa, tela submucosa, tunica muscularis, and tunica serosa—comprise the structure of the teleost digestive tube and all are present in the esophagus (Fig. 9A) (Harder 1975).

The tunica mucosa is stratified squamous epithelium, three to four cells thick, that rests atop a thick basement membrane (Fig. 9B). No lamina propria is present as it is replaced by the stratum compactum of the submucosa (Fig. 9A,B). Rostrally, taste buds occur in the distal portion of primary folds, whereas Type-A goblet cells are situated on the sides and at the bases of the folds. Centrally, 90 to 100% of the epithelium contains goblet cells and, as in the buccal cavity, these cells are overlain by squamous epithelium (Fig. 9F). Caudally, in the transitional area between esophagus and corpus ventriculi, the mucosal folds lengthen and gradually the epithelium changes to a columnar type. Fewer goblet cells and scattered rodlet cells, similar to those described by Flood et al. (1975) for the endothelium of the bulbus arteriosus in the goldfish, are pesent here (see Respiratory System, page 46).

The esophageal tela submucosa has two layers: a stratum compactum of dense connective tissue that supports the mucosa, and an underlying zone of areolar connective tissue. Arteries, veins, lymphatic ducts, blood cells, fibrocytes, fat cells, nerve fibers, coarse eosinophilic granular leukocytes, and lymphocytes compose the diverse cell population of the submucosa in the esophagus and throughout the alimentary tract. Lymphocytes are especially noticeable in association with the basal layer of the esophageal mucosa and the columnar epithelium of the stomach and intestines. Interfascicular connective tissue of the submucosa surrounds bundles of striated submucosal muscle, which occur appositionally in triangular-shaped cords that terminate in the anterior section of the corpus ventriculi (Fig. 9A,C). A thick outer layer of circular striated muscle composes the tunica muscularis, which is well vascularized (Fig. 9A). No muscularis mucosae exist in the esophagus and a tunica serosa is present only where the esophagus extends into the peritoneal cavity. The latter contains an underlying fibrous connective tissue band and an outer simple squamous epithelium. The serosal connective tissue band is wider in the esophagus than in any other part of the digestive tube. Rostrally, this band widens gradually changing into areolar connective tissue proximal to the pharynx. Large vagus nerve fibers are present throughout the serosa in the esophagus.

Foregut: Stomach

The gastric mucosa has two histologically distinct areas: the corpus ventriculi–gastric cecum region (fundic stomach) and the pars pylorica (pyloric stomach). Both show primary and secondary longitudinal folding of their mucous membranes. The corpus ventriculi has the thickest mucosa in the digestive tube. This mucosa consists of simple columnar epithelium with basal nuclei, simple tubular gastric glands, and a thin lamina propria; it has no goblet cells (Fig. 10A,B). This epithelium is continuous with that of the gastric cecum and pars pylorica (Fig. 10C,D). The columnar cells change to cuboidal cells in the neck

---

Figure 9. Esophagus of a 3-year-old striped bass.

A. Transverse section of the esophagus (formol sublimate; HPS). Bar = 87 μm.
B. Transverse section of the rostral esophagus (formol sublimate; HPS). Bar = 19 μm.
C. Transverse section of the mid-esophagus (formol sublimate; HPS). Bar = 348 μm.
D. Transverse section of the caudal esophagus (formol sublimate; HPS). Bar = 240 μm.
E. The esophageal mucosa (formol sublimate; HPS). Bar = 112 μm.
F. Type A goblet cells of esophageal mucosa (formol sublimate; HPS). Bar = 9.8 μm.

1 Areolar connective tissue
2 Basement membrane
3 Circular muscle layer (muscularis)
4 Esophageal goblet cells (Type A)
5 Esophageal stratum compactum
6 Longitudinal submucosal muscle
7 Mucosa
8 Primary folds
9 Secondary folds
10 Stratified squamous epithelium
11 Stratum germinativum
12 Submucosa
13 Tertiary folds

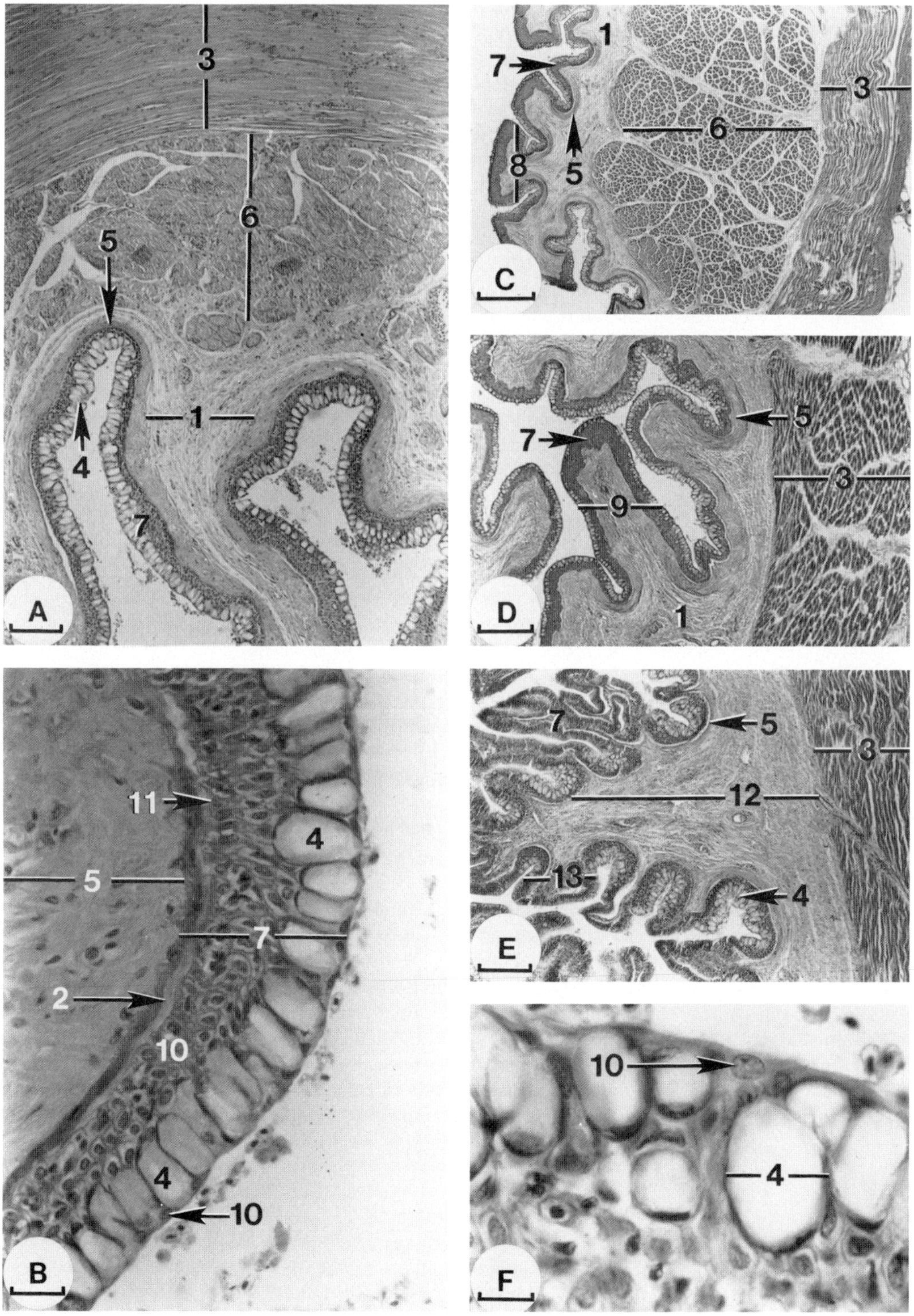

Figure 9

region of the underlying tubular gastric glands. Glandular cells uniformly contain acidophilic granules and, therefore, cannot be differentiated into parietal or chief cells. The lamina propria forms a thin vascularized network of connective tissue that supports the glands. No muscularis mucosae are present in the stomach. Migrating lymphocytes, coarse eosinophilic granular leukocytes, granulocytes, and rodlet cells, however, (Barber and Westermann 1975) commonly are found within this epithelial lining (Fig. 11B). In contrast, the mucosa of the pars pylorica contains no gastric glands and has a thin lamina propria (Fig. 11A,B). Here the complexity of the mucosal folds diminishes caudally toward the pyloric sphincter.

The submucosa of the corpus ventriculi and pars pylorica has two zones: a more vascularized outer zone of loose connective tissue containing a diverse cell population of lymphocytes, coarse eosinophilic granular leukocytes, fibrocytes, fat cells, arteries, veins, lymphatic ducts, and peripheral nerves; and an inner stratum compactum of dense collagenous connective tissue. Both zones extend into the primary folds of the mucous membrane. The stratum compactum is reduced in the thin-walled gastric cecum and is less dense in the pars pylorica.

The complete bi-layered tunica muscularis begins in the corpus ventriculi. Here the outer layer of striated circular muscle changes to smooth muscle and becomes the inner layer of the stomach muscularis (Fig. 10A,C). A new outer layer of longitudinal smooth muscle originates in this transitional zone. This bi-layer arrangement of the tunica muscularis is retained throughout the remainder of the digestive tube. Its inner circularis is well vascularized and separated in part from the longitudinale by the myenteric nerve plexus of Auerbach. In the corpus ventriculi the thickness of the circular layer is three times that of the longitudinal layer, whereas in the gastric cecum this ratio is closer to 10:1. Here the longitudinales form sweeping sheets that lie tangentially, rather than perpendicularly, against the circularis (Harder 1975). Both the original circularis and longitudinale are lost in the posterior gastric cecum, and a third layer, originating at the transitional zone between the corpus ventriculi and gastric cecum, replaces them. The muscularis is composed of an inner circular zone and an outer tangential zone of smooth muscle fibers. In the pars pylorica, and in particular at the pyloric sphincter, longitudinal submucosal smooth muscle bundles and fibers occur, resembling the muscularis mucosae of higher vertebrates. Here the circularis decreases to a thickness four to five times that of the longitudinale (Fig. 11A).

The tunica serosa of the stomach is a continuation of that covering the esophagus. It has the same simple squamous epithelium, but contains a thinner, underlying fibrous connective-tissue band.

Hindgut: Pyloric Ceca

The anterior intestine and its appendages, the pyloric ceca, originate immediately caudal to the pyloric sphincter. They differ histologically from the stomach by having decreased amounts of submucosal and muscular tissue and longer mucosal folds (Fig. 11C,D). Similarly, the columnar epithelial cells of the anterior intestines have a more prominent brush border than those of the stomach. In addition, Type-B goblet cells are present throughout the mucosa of both the pyloric ceca and intestines (Fig. 11E) (refer to page 32). The lamina propria of the pyloric ceca is highly vascularized and extends throughout the complex folds of the mucosa. Lymphocytes and coarse eosinophilic granular leukocytes also are prominent in both the mucosa and submucosa.

The muscularis is patterned after that of the intestines (inner circular muscle and outer longitudinal muscle): thin, with four times as much circular muscle as longitudinal muscle. Located between these two layers are ganglia of the plexus of Auerbach. The serosa again is simple squamous epithelium but it is absent in areas of the ceca

---

Figure 10. Stomach of a 3-year-old striped bass.

A. Transverse section of the corpus ventriculi (stomach) (Serra's; HPS). Bar = 240 μm.
B. Mucosa of the corpus ventriculi (Serra's; HPS). Bar = 19 μm.
C. Transverse section of the gastric cecum (Serra's; HPS). Bar = 240 μm.
D. Caudal region of the gastric cecum (Serra's; HPS). Bar = 34 μm.

1 Circular muscle layer
2 Columnar epithelial cells
3 Gastric glands
4 Lamina propria
5 Longitudinal muscle layer
6 Lumen of the corpus ventriculi
7 Muscularis
8 Submucosa
9 Veins

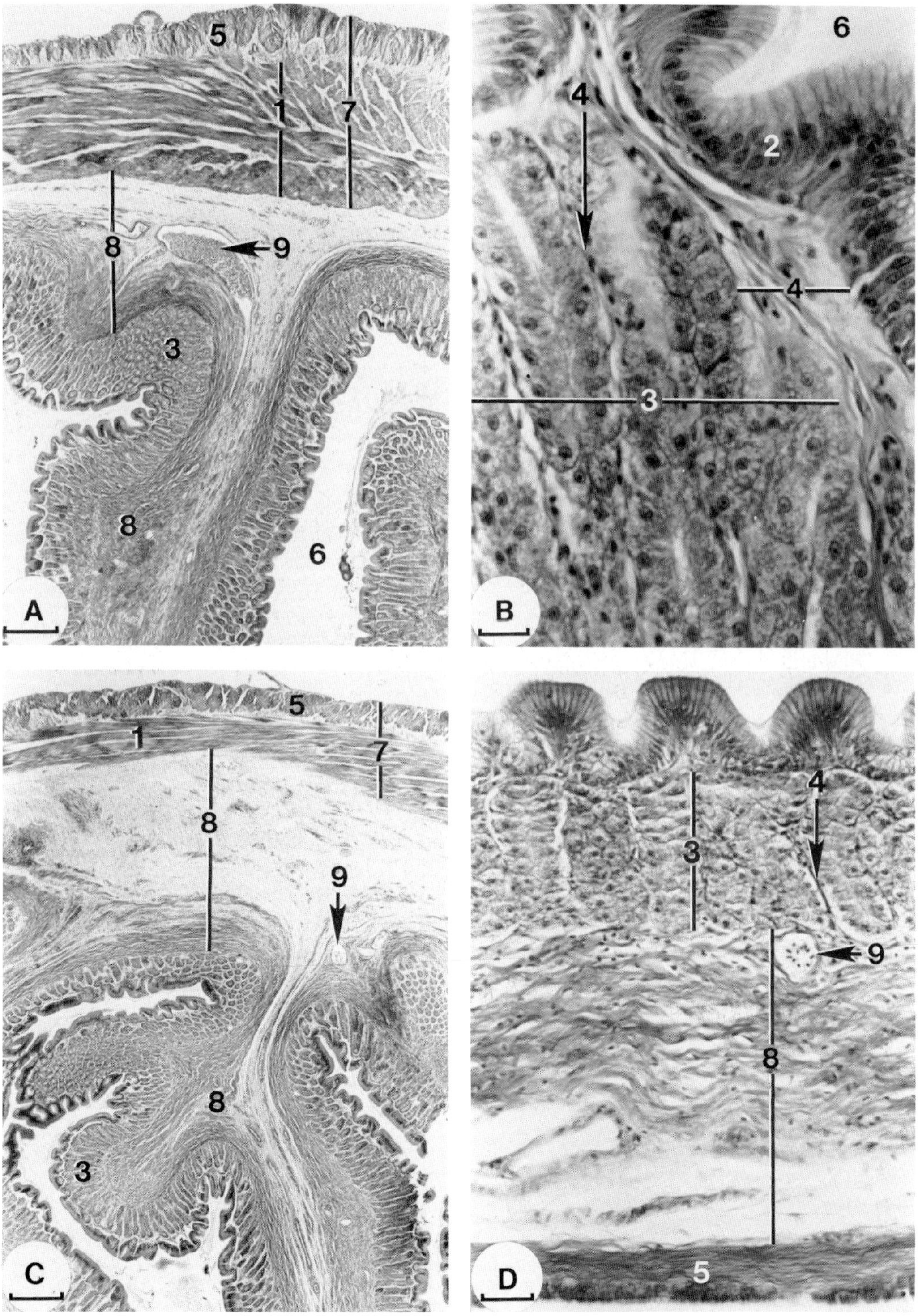

Figure 10

connected to the pars pylorica by mesenteries. In its place, loose connective tissue connects the longitudinal muscle layers of the pyloric stomach and ceca (Fig. 11C).

Hindgut: Anterior Intestine and Rectum

The anterior intestine and the rectum are difficult to separate grossly and histologically. The mucosa of both contain a vascular lamina propria and a simple columnar epithelium with Type-B goblet cells (Fig. 12A–D). The percentage of goblet cells in the mucosa varies, however, throughout the intestines—15% in the anterior intestine, 20% in most of the rectum, and up to 40% proximal to the anus. Differences also exist in the morphology of the mucosal folds. In the anterior intestine, the primary and secondary folds are long and complex, shortening toward the intestinal valve (Fig. 12E). The rectum has shorter primary and fewer secondary folds; both flatten near the anal pore (Figs. 12E, 13A). Here, goblet cells are all but absent from the mucosa where it merges with the integumental epithelium of the anal papilla (Fig. 13A). Rodlet cells are present in the columnar epithelium throughout the intestine (see Respiratory System, page 46).

The intestinal valve is the morphologic separation between anterior intestine and rectum. As noted above, it consists of a circular tissue flap, with a central opening, that is directed caudally within the rectal lumen (Fig. 12E). The mucosal and submucosal layers of the valve are continuous with those of the intestine proper; however, only the circular layer of the intestinal muscularis is present in the valve. It is discontinuous, being separated into parallel halves, one originating from the anterior muscularis and one from the rectal muscularis.

The intestinal submucosa (anterior and rectal) primarily differs from that found in the foregut by possessing denser connective-tissue elements and a greater population of coarse eosinophilic granular leukocytes. Similarly, the components of the muscularis (circularis, longitudinale, Auerbach's plexus) remain intact throughout the intestine, but their relative proportions change between the anterior and rectal sections. Specifically, the circularis increases in width to five or six times that of the longitudinale and Auerbach's nerve plexus is greatly enlarged. Proximal to the anus, the circularis terminates, whereas the longitudinale and myenteric plexuses merge with elements of the ventral body wall (Fig. 13B). Exocrine pancreatic tissue may be located in pockets within the intestinal muscularis where it surrounds exiting hepatic portal veins.

The teleost alimentary tract contains four autonomic nervous components to aid with muscular peristalsis and digestion: subserosal; myenteric or Auerbach's plexus; submucous; and subepithelial (Harder 1975; Wong and Tan 1981). Campbell and Gannon (1976) confirmed the adrenergic nature of these parasympathetic ganglia in brown and rainbow trout. In striped bass, only Auerbach's plexus is easily distinguished without the aid of special histochemical stains. This nerve plexus contains two morphologically distinct types of neurons: large Type-I neurons that possess large clear staining nuclei (often multiple) with a single, large nucleolus; and smaller Type-II neurons that contain smaller, more basophilic and more densely staining nuclei (Fig. 12F). In addition, Schwann cells, unmyelinated nerve fibers, and connective-tissue elements also are present in these plexuses. Burstock (1959) reported the presence of at least three histochemically distinct neurons in the brown trout myenteric plexus. Wong and Tan (1981), however, examined the ultrastructural components of the coral fish myenteric and submucus plexuses and only identified a single type of ganglial neuron. Further histochemical and ultrastructural examination is needed before similar

Figure 11. Digestive system of a 3-year-old striped bass.

A. Transverse section of the pars pylorica (formalin; HPS). Bar = 89 μm.
B. Mucosa of the pars pylorica (Serra's; HPS). Bar = 42 μm.
C. Common wall of two pyloric ceca (formalin; HPS). Bar = 203 μm.
D. Transverse section of a pyloric cecum (formalin; HPS). Bar = 231 μm.
E. Mucosa of the pyloric ceca (Serra's; HPS). Bar = 8.9 μm.

1 Blood vessel
2 Cecal villi
3 Cecal wall
4 Circular muscle layer
5 Columnar epithelium
6 Exocrine pancreatic tissue
7 Goblet cells (Type B)
8 Lamina propria
9 Longitudinal muscle layer
10 Mucosa
11 Muscularis
12 Red blood cells
13 Submucosa
14 Rodlet cells

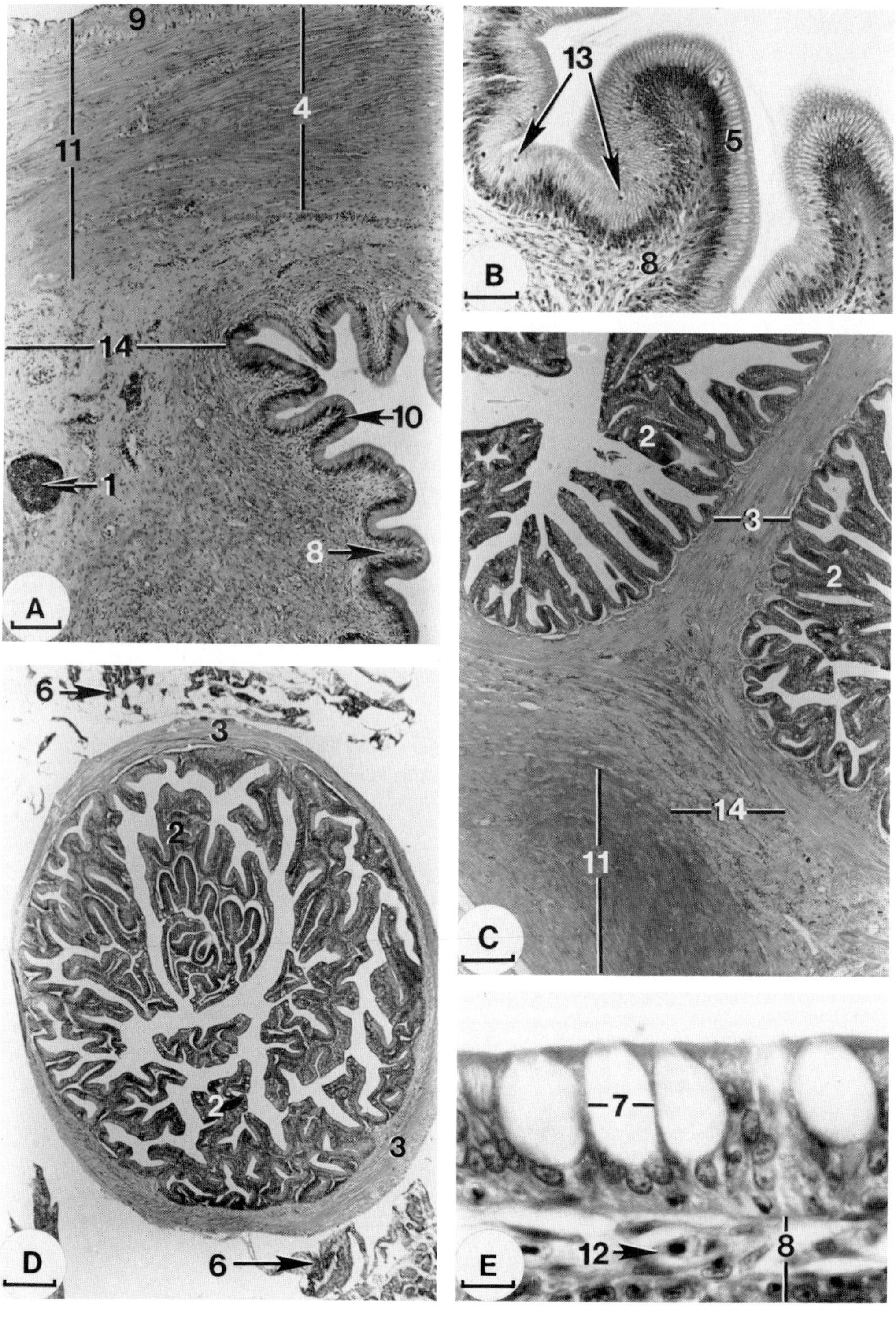

Figure 11

Table 2. *Alcian-blue (AB) and periodic-acid–Schiff (PAS) staining for mucosubstances in the alimentary tract of striped bass. Positive staining is indicated by +. HAS: hyaluronic acid and sialomucins; NM: neutral mucosubstances.*

Mucosal location	Cell type	Cell color	Probable mucosubstance	Fixative
Premaxillary jaw	Type-A goblet cell	AB+ (blue-black) PAS+ (magenta)	HAS NM	Formol sublimate Formol sublimate
Dentary jaw	Type-A goblet cell	AB+ PAS+	HAS NM	Formol sublimate
Tongue	Type-A goblet cell	AB+ PAS+	HAS NM	Formol sublimate
Pharyngeal	Type-A goblet cell	AB+ PAS+	HAS NM	Formol sublimate
Esophagus	Type-A goblet cell	AB+	HAS	Formol sublimate
Corpus ventriculi	Columnar epithelial cell	PAS+	NM	Serra's
Gastric cecum	Columnar epithelial cell	PAS+	NM	Serra's
Pars pylorica	Columnar epithelial cell	PAS+	NM	Serra's
Pyloric ceca	Type-B goblet cell	AB+	HAS	Serra's
Anterior intestine	Type-B goblet cell	AB+	HAS	Serra's
Intestinal valve	Type-B goblet cell	AB+	HAS	Serra's
Rectum	Type-B Goblet cell	AB+	HAS	Serra's
Anus	Type-B goblet cell	AB+	HAS	Serra's

comparisons can be made with striped bass nervous tissues.

The serosa of the anterior intestine and rectum is composed of a simple squamous epithelium. A thin fibrous connective-tissue layer separates it from the longitudinale. Caudally, the connective-tissue layer expands to surround the anus and the serosa becomes continuous with the lining of the peritoneal cavity.

Mucosubstances in the Alimentary Tract

Mucosubstances in the mucosa of the striped bass alimentary tract were screened by the alcian-blue–periodic acid–Schiff technique. Histological sections were made from the buccal cavity (premaxillary and dentary jaw elements), oral valve, tongue, pharyngeal pad, esophagus, corpus ventriculi, gastric cecum, pars pylorica, anterior intestine, pyloric ceca, intestinal valve, rectum, and anus (Table 2). The alcian-blue-positive substances (AB+), which stain dark blue, probably represent hyaluronic acid sulphomucins and sialomucins, whereas the periodic acid–Schiff-positive substances (PAS+), which stain magenta to red, probably represent neutral glycoproteins, according to Luna (1967) and Gona (1979).

The luminal epithelium of the mucosa that is associated with the premaxillary bone and oral valve contains approximately 50% goblet cells. These cells stain predominantly AB+. This observation agrees with that of Gona (1979) for the mucus-secreting cells in the oral valve of four belontoid fishes. The thin area associated with the basement membrane stains as a distinct PAS+ line. This structure is seen consistently throughout the alimentary tract and may indicate the presence

Figure 12. Intestine of a 3-year-old striped bass.

A. Transverse section of the anterior intestine (Serra's; HPS). Bar = 87 μm.
B. Intestinal mucosa (formol sublimate; H&E). Bar = 17 μm.
C. Transverse section of the rectal wall (Serra's; HPS). Bar = 62 μm.
D. Rectal mucosa (formalin; H&E). Bar = 43 μm.
E. Sagittal section of the intestinal valve (Serra's; HPS). Bar = 727 μm.
F. Auerbach's plexus in the rectum (Serra's; HPS). Bar = 21 μm.

1 Auerbach's plexus
2 Blood vessel
3 Circular muscle layer
4 Columnar epithelium
5 Goblet cells (Type B)
6 Hindgut (rectum)
7 Intestinal valve
8 Lamina propria
9 Longitudinal muscle layer
10 Midgut (anterior intestine)
11 Muscularis
12 Schwann cell
13 Serosa
14 Submucosa
15 Type I neuron
16 Type II neuron
17 Vein
18 Mucosal epithelium

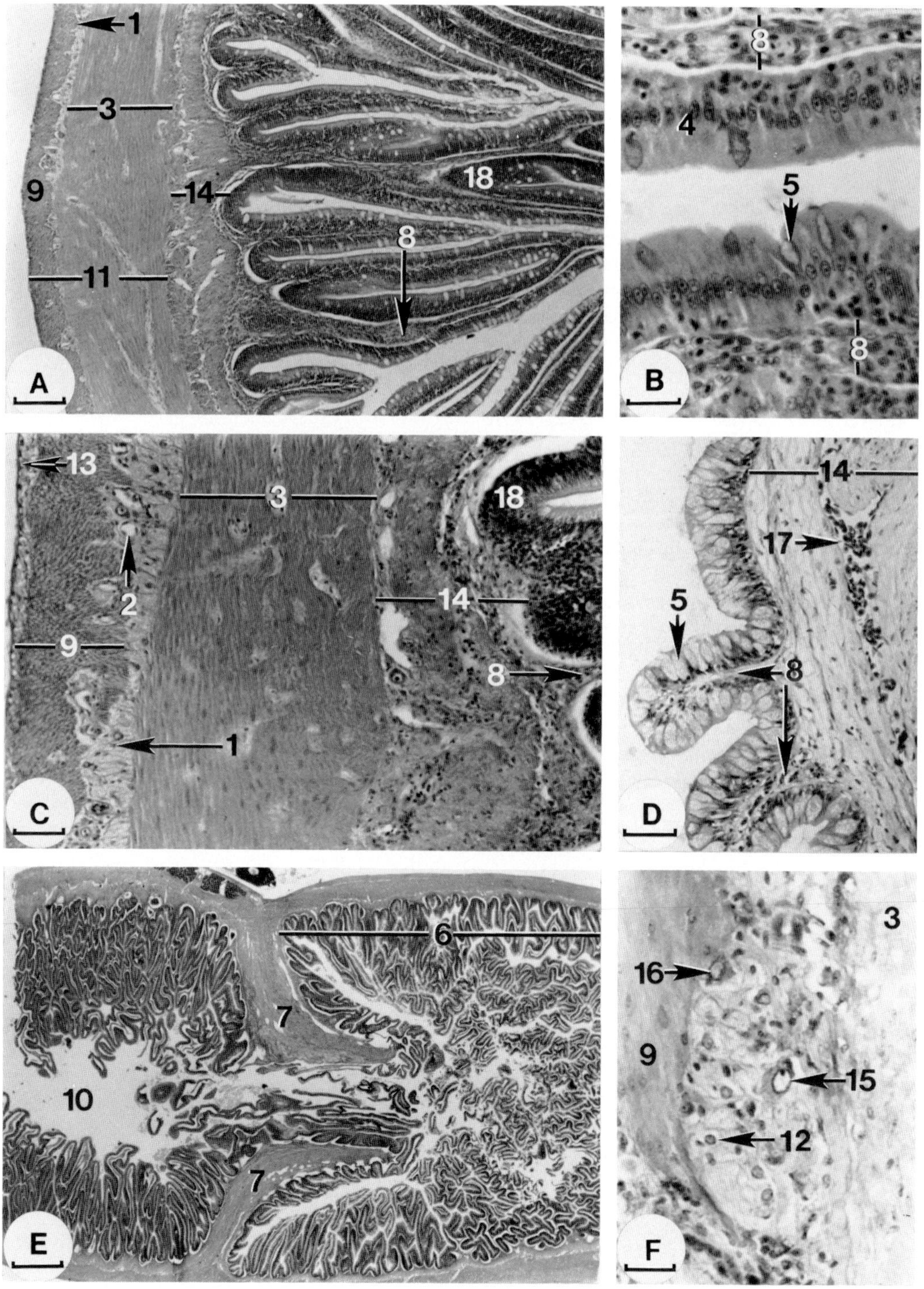
1
3
9
14
18
8
11
A
8
4
5
8
B
13
3
18
2
14
9
8
1
C
14
17
5
8
D
6
7
10
7
E
3
16
9
15
12
F

Figure 12

of actively deposited glycoproteins. Ham (1974) suggested that these glycoproteins constitute the basement membrane (Fig. 9B).

The mucosa of the lower-jaw dentary contains goblet cells that stain like those of the premaxillary area. Noteworthy is the increase of 50 to 80% in the number of goblet cells that line the cavities created by two oral flaps occurring luminally along the roof and base of the buccal cavity: that is, on both jaws. These flaps are continuous with the jaws on three sides (rostral, dextral, sinistral) having only their caudal edges unattached.

The tongue contains few goblet cells. Substantial numbers occur only in the mucosa associated with centrally or peripherally located teeth and along the basal attachment of the tongue to the buccal cavity. Similarly, the toothed area of the pharyngeal pad mucosa contains AB+ and PAS+ globlet cells in a 2:1 ratio (Plate 2E). The AB+ cells occur side by side as columnar cells and are located uniformly along both sides and into the crypts of the papillae. The PAS+ cells appear in a more random fashion, often between and below the AB+ cells or along the tips of the papillae.

The pattern described above for the occurrence of AB+ goblet cells is similar in the esophagus. There are more AB+ columnar goblet cells, however, occupying the tips of the papillae, and fewer PAS+ cells. Adjacent to the transitional zone between esophagus and corpus ventriculi, the goblet cells are confined to the crypts of the papillae. The histologic structure (round to oval with basally flattened nucleus) and staining quality (blue to blue-purple, representing sialomucins) of the esophageal mucous cells in striped bass are similar to those described for Type-A cells by Reifel and Travill (1977) for other teleosts.

A distinct break between esophagus and corpus ventriculi occurs, both in the cell type (stratified squamous to columnar) and in the mucoid-staining characteristics of the epithelium. No AB+ goblet cells are present in the stomach. The columnar cells there stain PAS+ in their apical cytoplasm. This quality is continuous throughout the epithelium of the gastric cecum and pars pylorica.

In the anterior intestine and pyloric ceca, the cytoplasm of the columnar epithelial cells does not stain PAS+; rather, AB+ goblet cells are present. This pattern is similar along the intestinal valve and rectum. In addition, a faint PAS+ area is present in the cytoplasm of the intestinal epithelium just below the microvilli. The number of goblet cells increases slightly in the rectum just anterior to the anus, where AB+ goblet cells predominate, but scattered PAS+ goblet cells also are present.

The goblet cells of the buccal cavity and esophagus in striped bass are histologically distinct from those of the intestines. In the former (which will be designated as Type A), the entire cytoplasm is filled with mucosubstances as described by Reifel and Travil (1977) (Fig. 9F). In the latter (which will be designated as Type B), the mucosubstances do not occupy more than one-half of the cytoplasm (Fig. 11E). In both Type-A and Type-B goblet cells, the nucleus is basally located.

Extramural Organs

The extramural organs of the striped bass include the gall bladder, pancreas, liver, and gas bladder. The gall bladder is situated within the fovea vesica biliaris (Harder 1975), the space created between the liver and anterior intestine. It is connected to the biliary system of the liver by the cystic duct and to the anterior intestine by the ductus choledochus. Bile produced in the liver can be stored within the gall bladder and later dispersed to the intestines via this duct (Fänge and Grove 1979).

Figure 13. Digestive system and extramural organs of striped bass.

A. Anal opening of the rectum, 3-month-old fish (formalin; H&E). Bar = 40 μm.
B. Junction of the rectum and the body wall, 3-year-old fish (formalin; HPS). Bar = 364 μm.
C. Gall bladder and pancreatic tissue, 3-year-old fish (formalin; AF). Bar = 270 μm.
D. Gall bladder epithelium, 3-year-old fish (formalin; PTAH). Bar = 9.4 μm.
E. Transverse section of the ductus choledochus, proximal to the gall bladder, 3-year-old fish (formalin; PTAH). Bar = 87 μm.

1 Anal opening
2 Body wall
3 Columnar epithelial cells
4 Endocrine pancreatic tissue
5 Epidermis
6 Exocrine pancreatic tissue
7 Fibrous connective tissue
8 Goblet cells
9 Hindgut (rectum)
10 Lumen of the gall bladder
11 Lumen of the rectum
12 Mesenteric fat
13 Mucosa
16 Muscularis
17 Submucosa
18 Wall of the gall bladder
19 Leukocytes

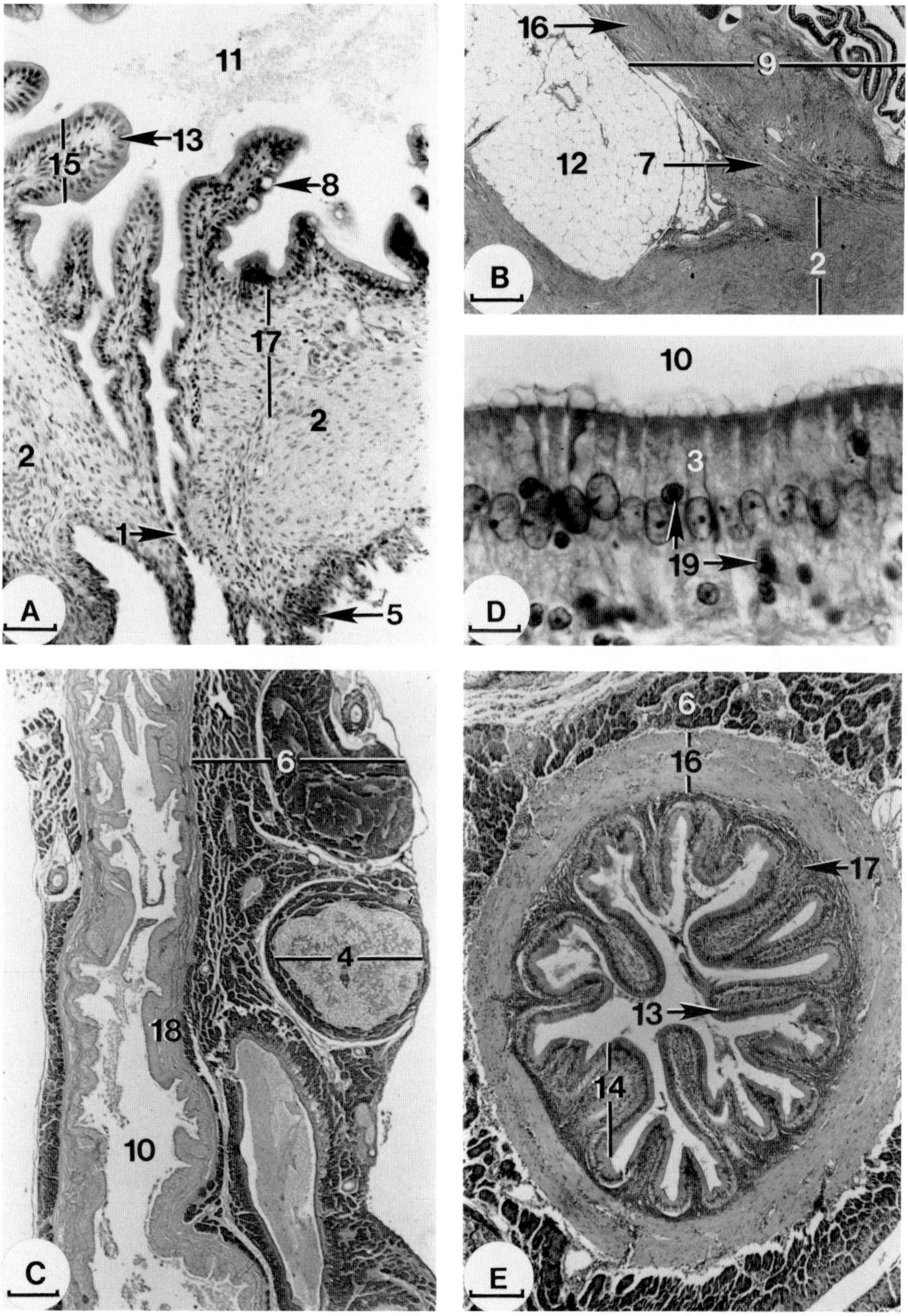

Figure 13

The striped bass has a diffuse pancreas that can be found scattered within the mesenteries and viscera in the peritoneal cavity (Khalilov 1966). Exocrine pancreatic tissue may surround the portal veins, from their origins beneath the tunica serosa of the intestines to their terminus within the liver. It is also located within mesenteric fat beneath the serosa at the gall bladder, and in connective tissue between the pyloric ceca. The endocrine pancreas occurs as a large principal islet and several smaller islets adjacent to the neck of the gall bladder (Fig. 13C). This endocrine gland is surrounded by exocrine pancreatic tissue and can be classified as a true Brockmann body (Brinn 1973) (see Endocrine System, page 92).

The liver is positioned centrally within the peritoneal cavity, caudal to the transverse septum, ventral to the esophagus, and ventrorostral to the corpus ventriculi and pars pylorica. It is U-shaped and conforms to the viscera and peritoneal cavity proper (Fig. 1). Blood enters the liver caudally from the intestines via the hepatic portal veins and exits rostrally through the hepatic veins to the sinus venosus. The liver primarily functions in the assimilation of nutritive substances, production of bile, detoxification, hematopoiesis, and destruction of red blood cells, and is by far the largest and most versatile of the metabolic organs (Harder 1975).

Although the gas bladder has no function associated directly with digestion in teleosts, a discussion of its histologic structure is included here because its tissues have a common embryologic origin with those of the alimentary canal (Hall 1924). Striped bass have a single-chambered euphysoclistous gas bladder (Harder 1975). This hydrostatic organ fills much of the dorsal peritoneal cavity extending the length of the trunk kidney (Dobbin 1941) (Fig. 1).

Gall Bladder

The gall bladder possesses the basic four-layer structure (mucosa, submucosa, muscularis, serosa) found in the alimentary tract (Chakrabarte et al. 1973). The mucosa is composed of columnar epithelium with centrally located nuclei (Fig. 13D). These cells generally appear more cuboidal when the gall bladder is distended. The submucosa contains dense connective tissue and the muscularis is composed of irregularly arranged sheets of smooth muscle. In the neck or proximal region of the gall bladder, exocrine pancreatic tissue, blood vessels, and nerve fibers are present between the muscularis and serosa (Fig. 13C). The distal region, however, lacks this layer of pancreatic tissue and contains a serosa that is separated from the muscularis by a thin layer of alveolar connective tissue.

The gall bladder primarily functions as a storage receptacle for bile produced by the liver. The bile is delivered to the anterior intestine via the ductus choledochus (Fig. 13E), which is connected to the common bile or cystic duct. These ducts also are composed of the same basic layers as the gall bladder and digestive tube: a mucosa of columnar epithelium; a longitudinally folded submucosal of loose connective tissue; a muscularis of smooth muscle; and a mesothelial serosa (Fig. 14A). The muscularis begins just prior to the emergence of the common bile duct from the liver.

Pancreas

The basic structure of the exocrine pancreas is consistent with that throughout the digestive system and extramural organs in striped bass. Two alveolar cell types are present here: columnar cell attached by their basal ends to the portal veins; and the typical pyrimidal acinar cells, that, in groups of five to eight, form lobular acini with central lumina (Fig. 14C,D). Each acinar cell has a centrally to basally located nucleus containing a larger central nucleolus. Zymogen granules are located in the apical ends of these cells (Leeson and Leeson 1970).

In striped bass, as in mammals (Fiore et al.

Figure 14. Extramural organs of a 3-year-old striped bass.

A. Wall of the ductus choledochus (formalin; HPS). Bar = 42 μm.
B. Ductus choledochus proximal of the anterior intestine (formalin; HPS). Bar = 209 μm.
C. Perivascular pancreatic tissue in liver (ethanol; H&E). Bar = 17 μm.
D. Macrophage aggregation in exocrine pancreatic tissue (Bouin's; H&E). Bar = 17 μm.

1 Acinar cells (pyramidal)
2 Acinus of the pancreas
3 Blood vessel
4 Columnar epithelium
5 Common pancreatic ducts
6 Connective tissue capsule
7 Ductus choledochus
8 Hepatic portal vein
9 Muscularis
10 Peripheral nerve
11 Red blood cells
12 Submucosa
13 Tissue macrophages
14 Vacuolated hepatocytes

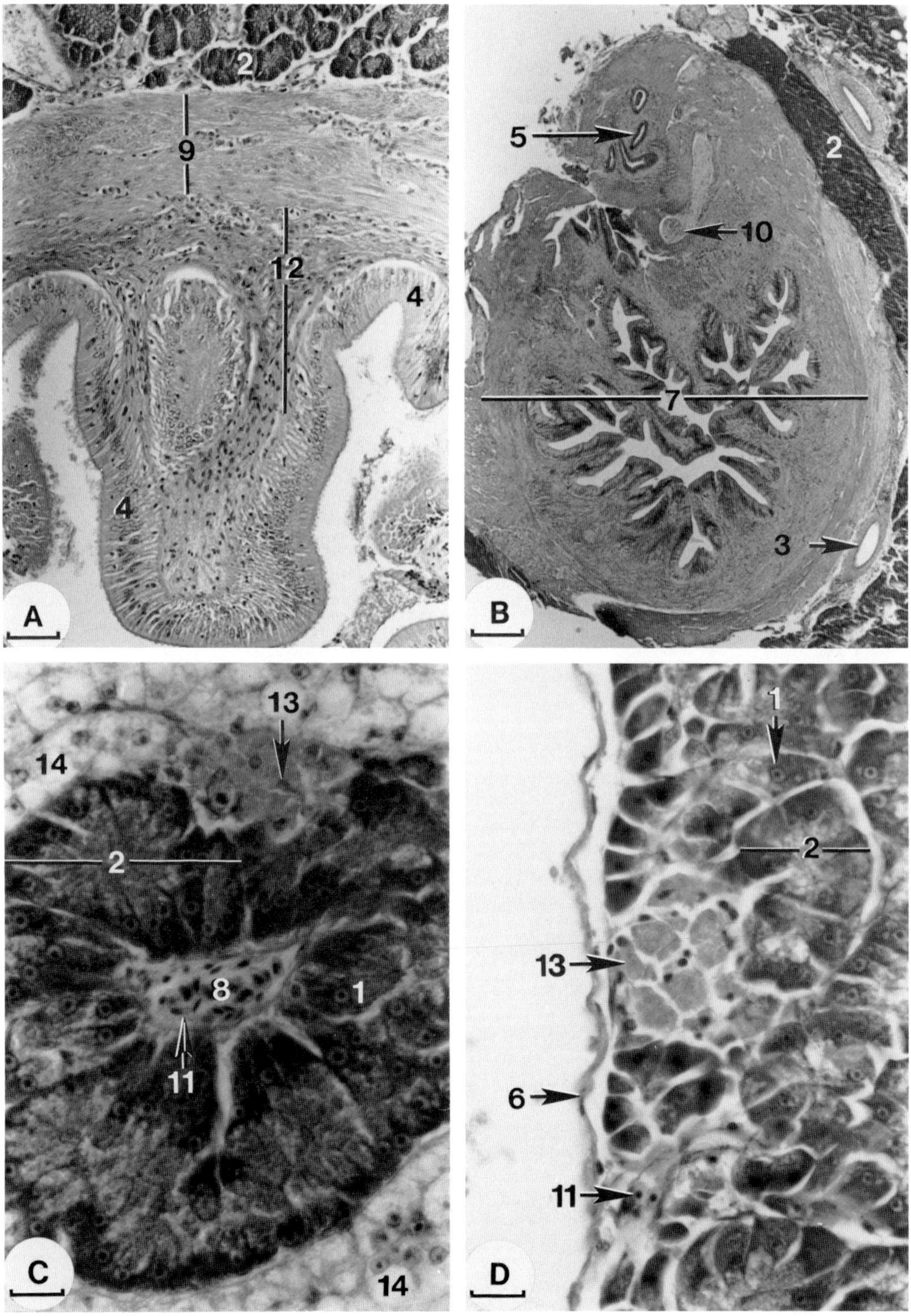

Figure 14

1973), centroacinar cells and intercalated ducts make up the primary delivery system for the pancreatic enzymes. These initial ducts combine to form larger interlobular pancreatic ducts (Fig. 15A) which, in turn, merge into the major pancreatic ducts that are contained within the connective tissue surrounding the epithelial lining of the ductus choledochus (Fig. 14B). The interrelated ducts are lined by cuboidal epithelium (Fig. 15A,B) that also can appear squamous (Fig. 15C) when the duct is distended. Interlobular ducts are distinguished from the above by a layer of dense connective tissue that surrounds their epithelial lining. These larger pancreatic ducts also have a mesothelial serosa when they occur extrapancreatically.

According to Fänge and Grove (1979), pancreatic secretions have not been thoroughly characterized in representative fish species. Several pancreatic enzymes, however, have been found in teleosts: proteases (trypsin, chymotrypsin, elastase, carboxypeptidase); amylase; chitinase; and lipases to mention a few. These enzymes, as in higher vertebrates, function in the digestive process occurring within the intestinal lumen.

Liver and Biliary System

The liver is encased within a fibroconnective tissue capsule and, unlike mammalian liver, it contains no distinct lobulation (Hinton et al. 1972), no apparent interlobular connective tissue stroma, and no typical portal triads. Rather, the most distinctive histological features of the liver include: exocrine pancreatic tissue that surrounds all of the portal veins in mature striped bass (Kristal 1946; Kendall and Hawkins 1975), and an anastomosing bilaminar meshwork of hepatocytes that comprises the basic functional hepatic units (Patt and Patt 1969) (Fig. 15D). The periportal pancreatic tissue forms a compound tubuloacinar gland and lies within a well vascularized fibroconnective tissue stroma (Fig. 15E).

Although true portal triads do not exist in the striped bass liver, bile ducts often are found in association with the exocrine pancreatic tissue surrounding portal veins (Fig. 15E). Hepatic arteries, however, seldom occur in combination with the above two structures and most often are isolated within the hepatic parenchyma, as are bile ducts (Fig. 15D,F).

Generally, hepatocytes appear as polyhedral cells with centrally located nuclei (Fig. 16A), but may demonstrate histological variability following extensive fat and glycogen storage (Woodhead 1977). When these cells contain large vacuoles of fat and many glycogen granules (Plate 3A,B), their nuclei and cytoplasm appear condensed and eccentrically positioned toward the nearest sinusoidal space (Fig. 16B,C). In addition to these structural components, hematopoietic tissue and accumulations of tissue macrophages may be present in the liver of adult fish (Fig. 16D).

In transverse section, liver sinusoids are bordered by five to eight, and separated by at least two, hepatocytes (Fig. 15E). These vascular spaces are lined by reticuloendothelial cells (Fig. 16C) that lie atop a fine network of reticular fibers (Plate 2F), similar to that found in channel catfish (Kendall and Hawkins 1975). Reticular fibers also are found along the central veins, portal veins, and pancreatic vasculature, and beneath the liver capsule (Plate 2F). Venous blood that enters the liver via the portal vein eventually flows through these sinusoids and collects in the central veins (Fig. 15D) before existing via the hepatic veins to the sinus venosus of the heart (Fig. 3A,B).

In the striped bass, no tubular lumina exist for the collection of bile, as is described for cyclostome liver by Patt and Patt (1969). Bile canaliculi are formed between adjacent hepatocytes (Fig. 16C) and are connected to larger bile ducts. As noted above, these ducts may occur within the parenchyma or in association with the exocrine

---

Figure 15. Extramural organs of a 3-year-old striped bass.

A. Interlobular pancreatic duct (formalin; PTAH). Bar = 18 μm.
B. Cuboidal epithelium of an interlobular pancreatic duct (Bouin's; HPS). Bar = 7.1 μm.
C. Intralobular pancreatic duct (Bouin's; H&E). Bar = 18 μm.
D. Liver (formalin; H&E). Bar = 615 μm.
E. Transverse section of a bile duct within pancreatic tissue (formalin; H&E). Bar = 44 μm.
F. Transverse section of a bile ductule in the liver parenchyma (formol sublimate; H&E). Bar = 9.7 μm.

1 Acinus of the pancreas
2 Bile duct (oblique section)
3 Central vein
4 Connective tissue layer
5 Cords of hepatocytes
6 Cuboidal epithelium
7 Hepatic portal vein
8 Hepatocytes
9 Pancreatic tissue
10 Red blood cells
11 Squamous epithelium

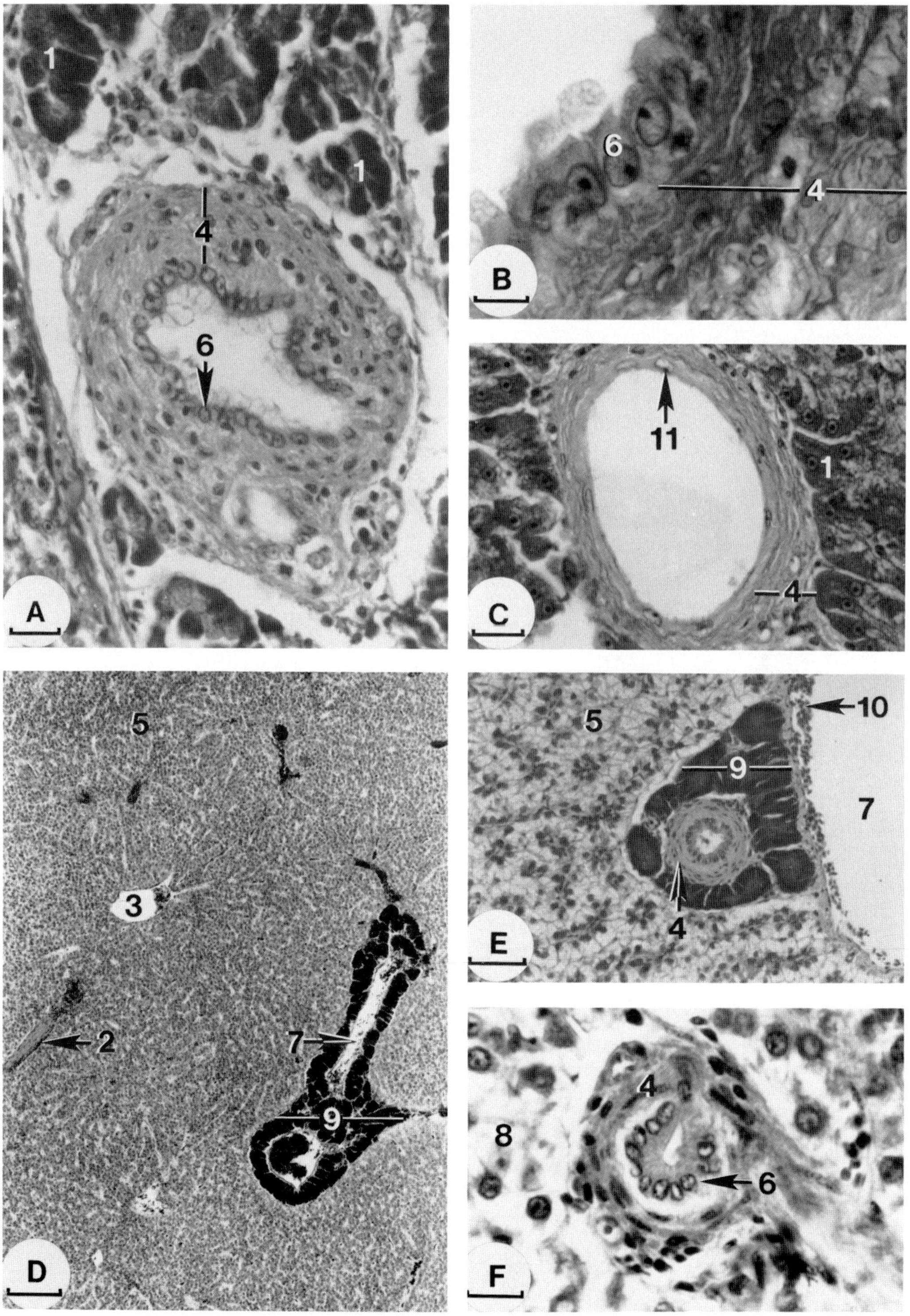

Figure 15

pancreas of the liver. They are lined by a low cuboidal epithelium and surrounded by a thin layer of fibrous connective tissue (Fig. 15E,F). The smaller bile ducts connect with the larger common bile duct before the latter emerges from the liver (see Gall Bladder, page 34). Fish bile is weakly alkaline and has a high sodium and low chloride concentration. It contains components similar to those of higher vertebrates: bile salts; cholesterol; phospholipids; bile pigments; organic anions; glycoproteins; and inorganic ions. All are important to proper micelle formation and lipid digestion in fish (Fänge and Grove 1979).

Gas Bladder

The striped bass has a well-developed gas gland and rete mirabile. The rete mirabile appears as a vascularization and enlargement of the rostroventral bladder wall, and has several layers (Fänge 1953): the serosa or tunica externa; a compact fibrous layer or tunica fibrosa; a muscularis; and an inner epithelial layer or tunica interna (Fig. 16E). In other regions of the gas bladder, the wall is thinner and less complex, lacking the rete mirabile.

The serosa is the peritoneal layer that covers the ventral surface of the gas bladder. It is very thin, consisting of an epithelial layer, connective tissue, blood vessels, and nerve fibers. Conversely, the tunica fibrosa forms a thickened collagenous connective-tissue layer that is bordered on its inside by a well-vascularized and innervated muscularis of smooth muscle bundles. Between the muscularis and submucosa is a layer of pigmented cells (Fig. 16E). Wittenberg et al. (1980) described this region in several deep sea fishes as possessing overlapping, nucleated, circular platelets containing pigments that may help resist the outward diffusion of gases. Inside this pigmented layer, a submucosa of loose connective tissue forms a major portion of the rete mirabile wall. The intricate capillary system of the rete is intimately associated with the cuboidal glandular epithelium of the tunica interna (Fig. 16F), which can range from one to several layers. The rete mirabile, like the choroid body of the eye (page 86), forms a countercurrent capillary system that enhances the quantity of gases (primarily oxygen) available to the epithelial component of the gas bladder, thereby allowing these gases to be concentrated within the gas bladder. In many euphysoclistrous fish, concentrated gases exit the bladder via resorption through a specialized oval, located in the dorsorostral region. No oval was apparent in the striped bass examined. This, however, does not rule out the possibility of such a capillary network in gas bladder of this species. Both secretion and resorption of gases by the teleost gas bladder are controlled by the autonomic nervous system (McLean and Nilsson 1981).

Reyer (1977) and Ross (1979) attributed several functions to the gas bladder in teleosts: hydrostatic equilibrium; respiration; sound production and sound intensification; and perception of oscillations in pressure. Harder (1975), however, suggested that the primary role is to serve as a sensory apparatus that provides information concerning the vertical component of the fish's swimming motion, but he provided little evidence for this function.

Figure 16. Extramural organs of a 3-year-old striped bass.

- **A.** Nonvacuolated hepatocytes of the liver (formalin; H&E). Bar = 9.2 μm.
- **B.** A central vein in the liver (formalin; H&E). Bar = 46 μm.
- **C.** Transverse section of a liver sinusoid surrounded by vacuolated liver parenchyma (formalin; H&E). Bar = 8.9 μm.
- **D.** An aggregation of tissue macrophages in the liver (formalin; H&E). Bar = 19 μm.
- **E.** Transverse section of the gas bladder wall (formol sublimate; H&E). Bar = 88 μm.
- **F.** Rete mirabile of the gass bladder (formol sublimate; HPS). Bar = 46 μm.

1 Bile canaliculus
2 Blood vessel
3 Central vein
4 Compact fibrous layer (tunica fibrosa)
5 Cords of hepatocytes
6 Endothelial cell
7 Gas gland epithelium (tunica interna)
8 Hepatocytes
9 Loose connective tissue (tunica interna)
10 Lumen of gas bladder
11 Muscularis
12 Peripheral nerve
13 Pigmented cell layer
14 Red blood cells
15 Serosa (tunica externa)
16 Tissue macrophages

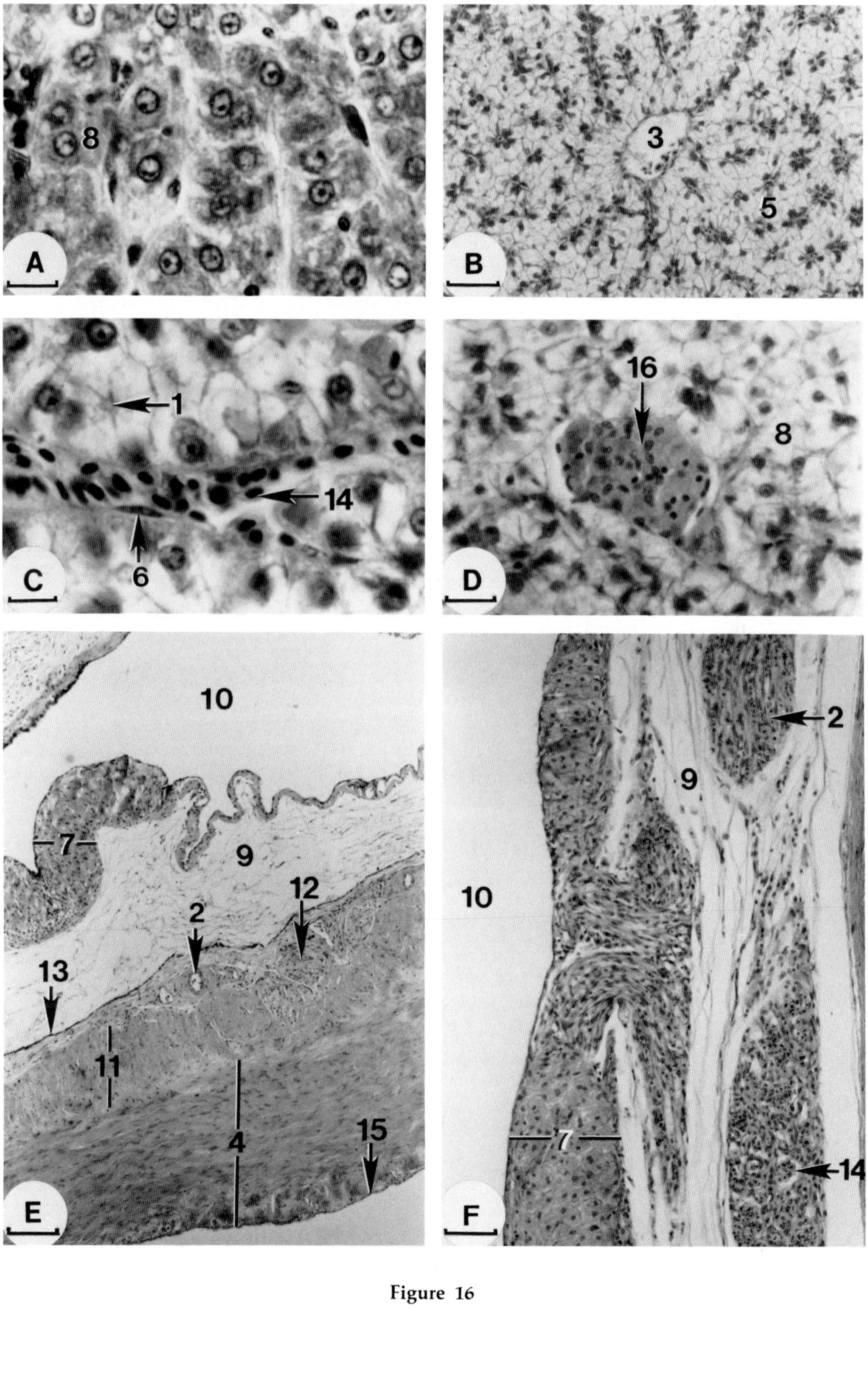

Figure 16

Respiratory System

Teleosts obtain oxygen from water by simple diffusion through gills. Striped bass have four pairs of gills, each of which is located along the caudolateral edges of the bilateral hypo-, cerato-, epi-, and pharyngobranchial bones of the gill arches (Harder 1975). These arches are situated within the pharyngeal cavity and extend from the floor to the roof along the lateral margins of the cavity. They are enclosed beneath the opercular or gill covers, which regulate water flow and protect the gills.

Each gill is made up of filaments or primary lamellae (Fig. 17A,B) arranged in double rows (holobranchiae) along the arch bones. According to Harder (1975) filaments from each succeeding holobranchia mesh with one another, forming a latticework through which the water from the oral cavity is forced to pass. This was not confirmed in striped bass. Secondary gill lamellae originate from the filaments and are perpendicular to the inferior and superior margins of each filament. Each secondary lamella contains a thin-walled gill sinusoid, and it is here that oxygen from the water diffuses into the blood. Gill rakers are located along the gill arches opposite the primary lamellae (Fig. 17C). They are constructed of acellular or mixed bone and covered by mucosal epithelium and acrodont teeth. The gill rakers are reduced to knobs on all but the most rostral pair of arches. This type of arrangement is termed biserial-dimorphic-monacanth, according to Harder (1975). Gill rakers help in the acquisition of food particles and protection of the gill filaments.

The gills function in respiration, excretion, and osmoregulation (Laurent and Dunel 1978) by means of sinusoids that allow for the continuous exchange of respiratory gases like oxygen and soluble metabolic waste such as carbon dioxide and ammonia. In addition, the respiratory epithelium of the secondary lamellae contains specialized chloride cells, or ionocytes, that assist with osmoregulation by excreting chloride, potassium, and sodium ions (Harder 1975). Chloride cells are most evident histologically in euryhaline species, such as the striped bass, during transitional periods between fresh and salt water (Fearnhead and Fabion 1971; Kikuchi 1977).

Respiratory Circulation

The striped bass gill possesses dual arterial pathways similar to those described by Laurent and Dunel (1976) for rainbow trout and yellow perch. They include an arterioarterial pathway that functions in respiration and an arteriovenous pathway that nourishes the gill arch and lamellar tissues. Blood exiting the heart flows via the ventral aorta to the four pairs of afferent branchial arteris. These arteries proceed up into each of the gill arches proximal to the primary lamellae (Fig. 17A,C,D). Blood moves from them into the afferent primary arteries, one of which runs along a groove in the cartilaginous gill ray of each filament (Fig. 17B). The sinusoids of the secondary lamellae branch off the afferent primary arteries (Fig. 18A). Blood flow in the sinusoids is counter to that of the respiratory water, thereby maximizing the amount of oxygen it can extract (Harder 1975). From the sinusoids, blood moves into the efferent

---

Figure 17. Gill of a 3-year-old striped bass.

A. Transverse section of a gill arch (Bouin's; HPS). Bar = 407 μm.
B. Filaments and secondary lamellase of a gill (formol sublimate; H&E). Bar = 89 μm.
C. Sagittal section of a gill arch and gill raker (Bouin's; HPS). Bar = 245 μm.
D. Enlargement from **A** showing blood vessels of the gill arch (Bouin's; HPS). Bar = 80 μm.

1 Acellular bone of gill arch
2 Adipose tissue
3 Afferent branchial artery
4 Capillaries
5 Cartilage of the gill filament
6 Central venus sinus
7 Efferent branchial artery
8 Gill arch spongy bone (arcus branchiales)
9 Gill filament
10 Gill raker (branchictenia, branchiospinae)
11 Nutritional blood vessel (branchial vein)
12 Peripheral nerve
13 Pharyngeal teeth
14 Secondary lamellae
15 Transverse septum

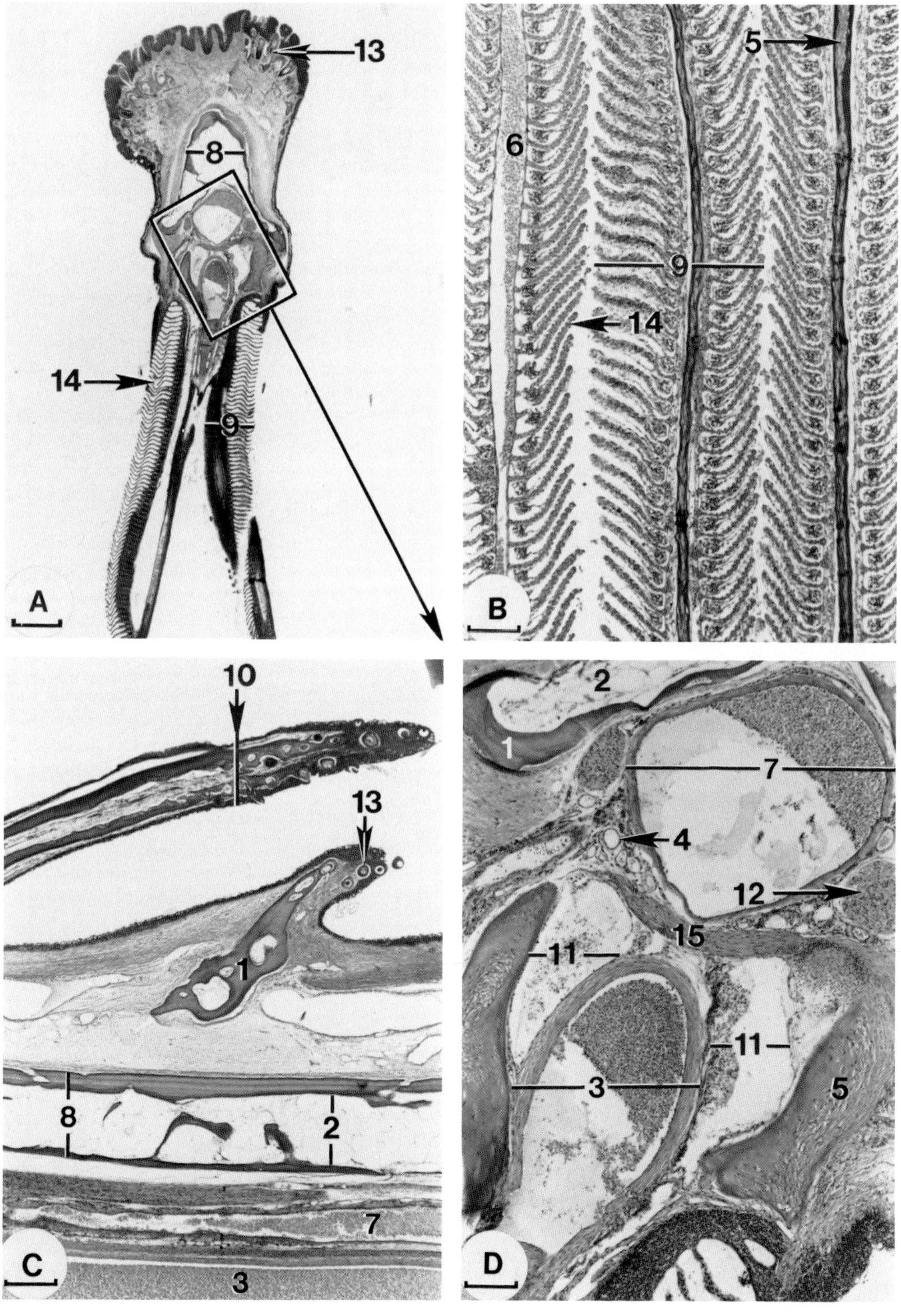

Figure 17

primary arteries located on the opposite sides of the filaments. At this point, the blood may either continue down the efferent primary artery to the efferent branchial artery or it can be shunted via small veins to the central venous sinus of the filament (Fig. 17B). The sinus occupies the core of the filaments and lies between the cartilage of the gill ray and the efferent primary artery. The central venous sinus connects with the branchial veins of the gill arch via small veins that run parallel to the afferent primary arteries of each filament. The branchial veins are lateral to the afferent branchial artery between the base of the gill rays and the transverse septum of the arch (Fig. 17D). These veins, together with others located in the submucosa of the gill arch, empty into the efferent branchial artery. Blood shunted from the efferent primary arteries to the efferent branchial artery is the source of oxygen to both the body and the arteriovenous system within the arch.

Oxygenated blood from the efferent branchial artery may move via small arteries to the tissues of the gill arch or directly to the central venous sinus of the primary lamellae. Subsequently, venous blood from the entire arch returns to the efferent branchial artery before exiting the gill (Fig. 17A,D). All of the circulatory pathways in the gill are innervated by branches of cranial nerves IX and X (glossopharyngeal and vagus, respectively) (Fig. 17D). According to Smith and Jones (1978) and Daxboeck and Holeton (1978), regulation of the respiratory rates or blood flow through the gills is accomplished with the help of oxygen receptors in some teleosts. These receptors are located superficially along the dorsal region of the first gill arch in rainbow trout and are also innervated by branches of cranial nerves IX and X. It is believed that stimuli from the oxygen receptors alter heart rate, ventilatory rate, and possibly other circulatory responses to changing ambient oxygen concentrations. The presence of similar receptors was not investigated in the striped bass.

Gill Arches

The cellular constituents of the gill arches are basically continuations of the ventral aorta, the buccal mucosal lining, and the skeletal elements of the striped bass cranium. With the exception of the branchial arteries, the walls of the other gill blood vessels are significantly reduced; the afferent primary artery walls contain only endothelial cells where they parallel the gill rays into the filaments. Conversely, the afferent branchial artery wall has more smooth muscle than any other blood vessel in the gill (Fig. 17D).

The epithelium covering the gill arches is continuous with both the mucosa of the buccal cavity and the epithelium of the gill filaments. It contains taste buds, mucous cells, and acrodont teeth (Fig. 17A,C). Along the rostral edge of each arch, the underlying submucosa is enlarged and contains numerous nonrespiratory blood vessels. Laterally along the arch, the submucosa is reduced to a few layers of dense connective tissue and some striated muscle bundles. According to Harder (1975) and Lagler et al. (1977), abductor muscle bundles occur along the outer lateral gill arch between the base of the gill ray and the bone of the gill arch in bony fish like striped bass. The paired adductor muscles, however, are located between hemibranchiae and cross over each other. Both of these muscle bundles help to hold the gill in a favorable position for respiration.

The composition of the gill arch bones and gill ray cartilage changes with the age of striped bass. In age-0 fish, a larger percentage of the specialized gill cartilage is present in both of these skeletal structures (Fig. 17D). Adult fish have reduced

---

Figure 18. Gill of a 3-year-old striped bass.

A. Secondary lamellae of the gill (gluteraldehyde; TB). Bar = 26 μm.
B. Enlargement from **A**, base of secondary gill lamellae (gluteraldehyde; TB). Bar = 9 μm.
C. Tip of secondary gill lamella (gluteraldehyde; TB). Bar = 10 μm.
D. Electron micrograph of a pillar cell in a secondary gill lamellae (gluteraldehyde; UALC). Bar = 0.6 μm.
E. Electron micrograph of a mucous cell in a secondary gill lamella (gluteraldehyde; UALC). Bar = 0.55 μm.
F. Electron micrograph of a chloride cell at the base of a secondary gill lamella (gluteraldehyde; UALC). Bar = 2.3 μm.

1 Arteriole space
2 Chloride cell of gill
3 Cytoplasmic mucous vacuole
4 Endoplasmic reticulum (cytoplasmic tubules)
5 Epithelial cell
6 Mitochondria
7 Mucous cell
8 Nucleus
9 Pillar cell
10 Red blood cells
11 Rodlet cell
12 Secondary gill lamella

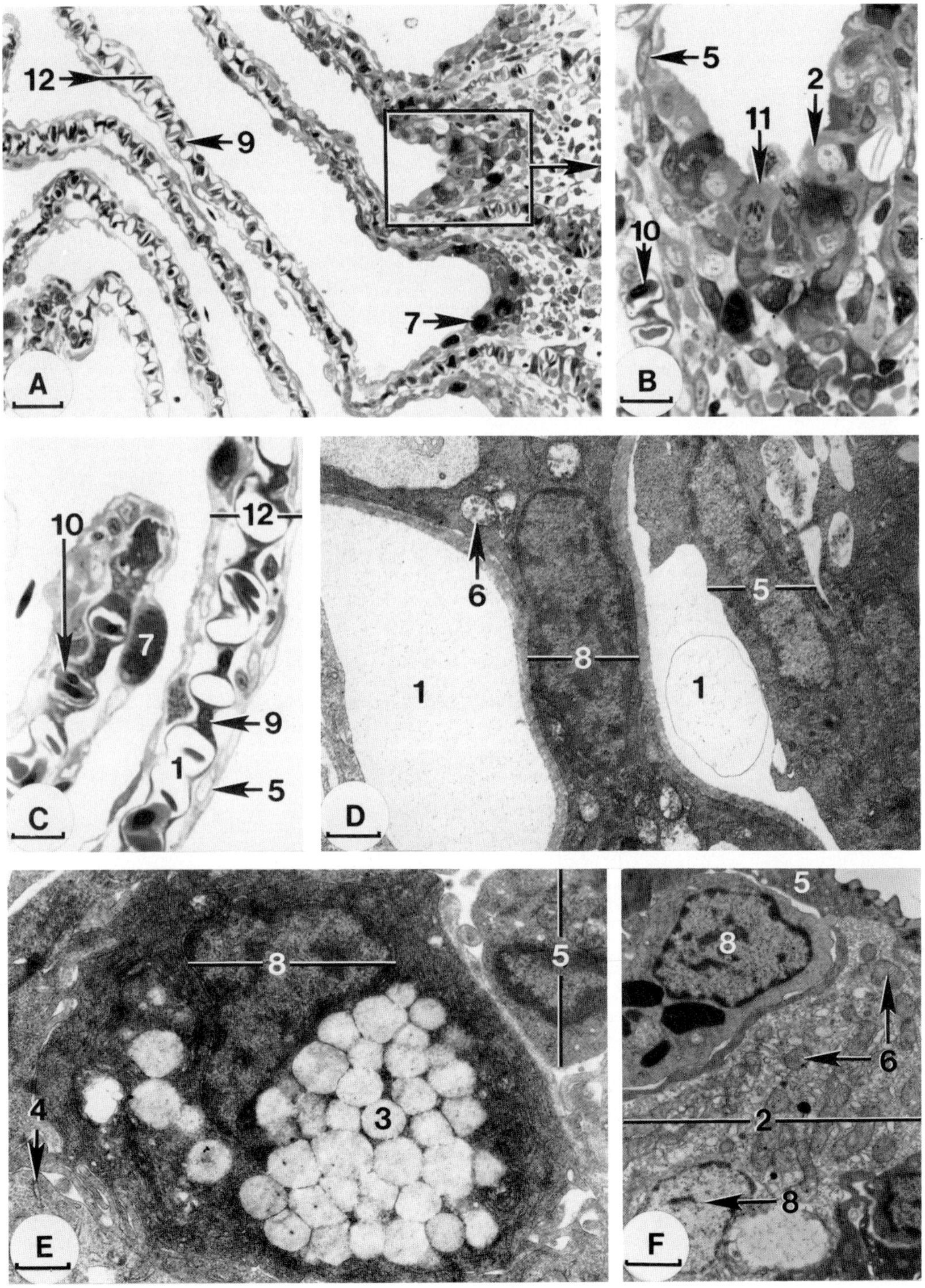

Figure 18

cartilaginous elements in the arch bones but not the gill rays. Similarly, the arch and gill rakers are composed of mixed bone best distinguished by its central adipose element and peripheral acellular element (Fig. 17C,D) (see Skeletal System, page 68).

Gill Lamellae

In addition to the blood vessels and cartilaginous gill rays described above, the primary lamellae (filaments) contain melanocytes, lymphocytes, macrophages, coarse eosinophilic granular leukocytes, endothelial cells, and epithelial cells. The secondary lamellae have mucous cells, rodlet cells, and chloride cells enclosed beneath an overlapping stratified squamous epithelium that is most prominent between the lamellae and at the tips or bases of the filaments (Fig. 18A,B). The primary lamellae serve more for support of the secondary lamellae than for respiration.

The secondary lamellae have an external layer of overlapping or interdigitating squamous epithelium (Fig. 18C) that is supported by a basement membrane and a thin layer of connective tissue (Anderson and Mitchum 1974). Bauer (1973) noted that the respiratory epithelium in striped bass held in sea water appeared irregular, whereas that from freshwater fish was smooth. Contractile pillar cells separate one side of a secondary lamella from the other (Fig. 18C). They contain abundant mitochondria (Fig. 18D) and a fine fibrous cytoplasm. It is generally accepted that the upper and lower margin of the pillar cells extend into interconnecting flanges that run parallel to the external epithelium (Hughes and Grimstone 1965; Grizzle and Rogers 1976; Roberts 1978). In striped bass, flanges and scattered endothelial cells delimit an extensive blood sinusoid system between adjacent pillar cells, where actual oxygen diffusion occurs. Roberts (1978) suggested that the blood flow through the sinusoids may be regulated by acetylcholine activation of the contractile fibers in the pillar cells. Mucous cells also occur in the space between the respiratory epithelium and the pillar-cell flanges (Gona 1979). These cells have eccentrically placed nuclei and large cytoplasmic mucous vacuoles (Fig. 18E).

The chloride cells or ionocytes of the gill lamellae are the primary osmoregulatory cells of fishes (Kirschner 1977). In striped bass sampled from sea water, the chloride cells contain large basal nuclei, numerous cytoplasmic vesicles, and mitochondria with enlarged separated cristae (Figs. 18F, 19A). An extensive network of intracytoplasmic tubules, which connects with the lateral and basal cell membranes, also is present (Kikuchi 1977; Schwerdtfeger and Bereiter-Hahn 1978). Bauer (1973) noted that a tubular labyrinth is present that allows electrolytes to move from the blood to the teleost chloride cells. This tubular system is composed of smooth endoplasmic reticulum and extends from both the blood vessel lumen and the chloride cells to an expanded intercellular space surrounding the vascular tissue of the respiratory lamellae. In some marine teleosts, apical crypts occur on the exposed surfaces of chloride cells, and allow for the release of ions to the environment. In contrast, chloride cells of fish held in fresh water contained microvilli on their free surfaces.

Figure 19. Gills and pseudobranchiae of striped bass.

A. Electron micrograph of a chloride cell located at the base of a secondary gill lamella, 3-year-old fish (gluteraldehyde UALC). Bar = 0.35 μm.
B. Electron micrograph of a rodlet cell (oblique section) in a secondary gill lamella, 3-year-old fish (gluteraldehyde; UALC). Bar = 0.74 μm.
C. Electron micrograph of a rodlet cell (transverse section) in a secondary gill lamella, 3-year-old fish (gluteraldehyde; UALC). Bar = 0.74 μm.
D. Transverse section through the pseudobranch, 3-month-old fish (Bouin's; H&E). Bar = 89 μm.
E. Lamella of the pseudobranch, 3-week-old fish (formalin; H&E). Bar = 5.6 μm.

1 Blood vessel
2 Cytoplasmic mucous vacuole
3 Cytoplasmic vesicle
4 Electron-dense granule
5 Endoplasmic reticulum (cytoplasmic tubules)
6 Epithelial cell
7 Fibrous capsule
8 Gill cavity
9 Glandular pseudobranch cell
10 Hyaline cartilage
11 Lymph vessel
12 Membrane-bound vesicle
13 Mitochondria
14 Nucleus
15 Oral mucosa
16 Pseudobranch lamellae
17 Red blood cells
18 Rodlets
19 Skeletal muscle bundles

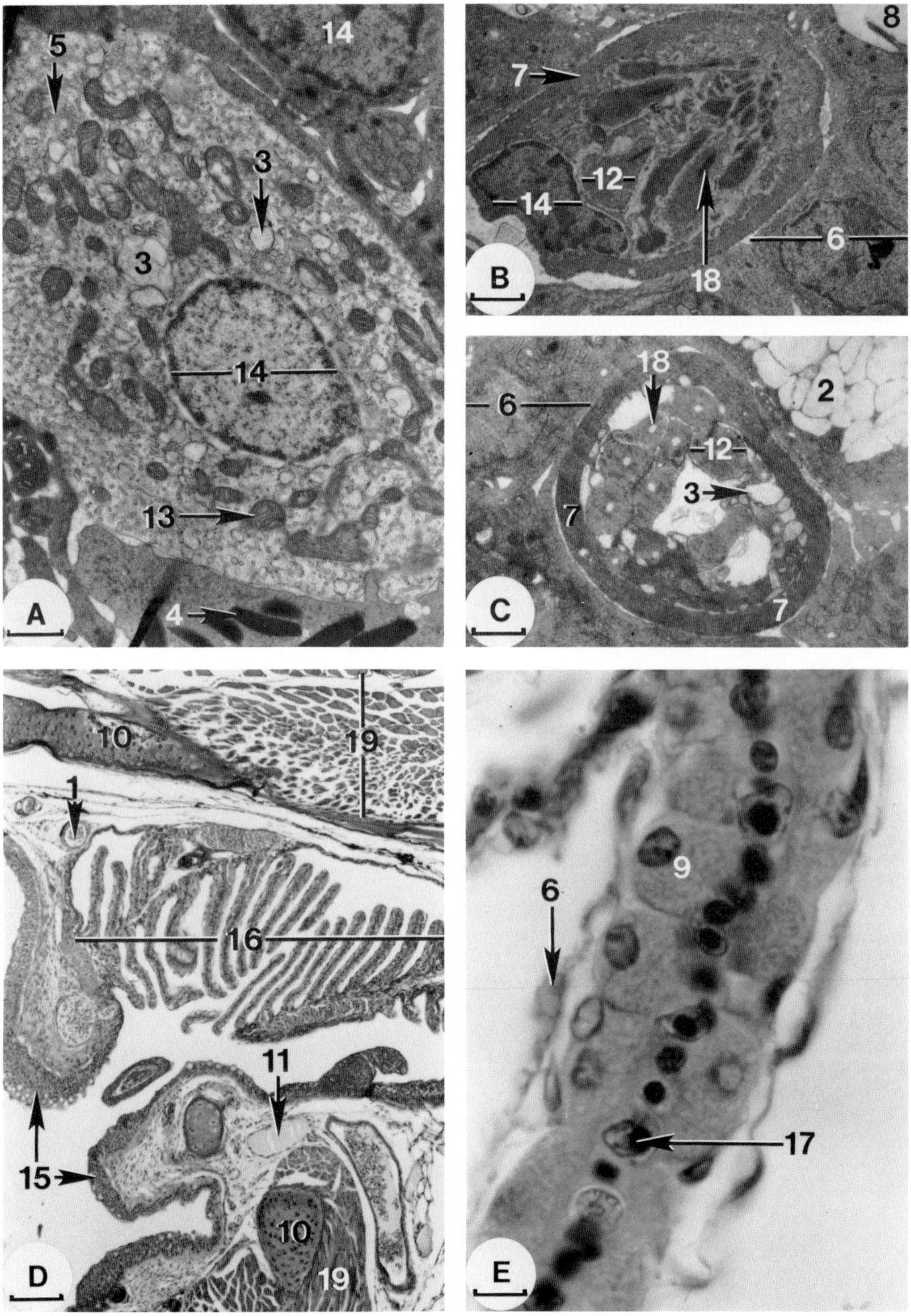
5
3
3
14
14
13
4
A
8
7
12
14
18
6
B
18
6
2
12
3
7
7
C
10
19
1
16
11
15
10
19
D
9
6
17
E

Figure 19

In the gills, rodlet cells occurred primarily at the base of the secondary lamellae of striped bass examined for this study, (Fig. 18B) and were oriented perpendicularly to the lamellar epithelium. Rodlet cells contain all of the basic organelles described by Morrison and Odense (1978): basally placed nucleus; thick fibrous capsule; cytoplasmic vesicles; and membrane bound vesicles (Fig. 19B,C). Within the latter vesicles are the crystalline rodlets for which these cells are named.

Rodlet cells occur in many epithelial tissues of fishes: gill lamellae; pseudobranchiae; kidney tubules; pancreatic and biliary ducts; intestinal mucosa; and olfactory epithelium, to name a few. Presently, debate continues over their origin and function. Are these cells secretory or parasitic in nature? Flood et al. (1975) concluded, after ultrastructure studies, that rodlet cells behave as foreign bodies. Barber and Westermann (1975) suggested that this cell may represent a stage in the life history of a parasite. Grünberg and Hager (1978) contend that it is not a parasite. An extensive literature review on this debate has been compiled by Morrison and Odense (1978), who presented electron micrographs and histochemical evidence to support the contention that this is a normal cell of fish. They believe that the cell produces a neutral glycoprotein, which could have either a similar function to the mucin secreted by goblet cells or an enzymatic one. Recently, Barber et al. (1979) reaffirmed their contention that rodlet cells are parasites or infective agents. This observation was supported by Mayberry et al. (1979) who classified the rodlet cell as the sporazoan *Rhabdospora thelohani,* a member of the Apicomplexa. Mattey et al. (1979), however, presented contradictory evidence that suggests this cell is indeed similar to, or complementary to, mucous cells, whose secretions may be involved in pH control.

In striped bass, rodlet cells primarily occur in the gill lamellae (Figs. 18B, 19B,C), olfactory epithelium (Fig. 34F), intestinal mucosa, pancreatic and bile-duct epithelia, mesenteries, kidney tubules (Fig. 21B,C), urinary-bladder epithelium, and lateral-line organs. By light microscopy, these cells appear bulb-shaped, stain eosinophilically, and often seem to occur intracellularly. In accordance with the findings of Mattey et al. (1979) for the bass *Dicentranchus labrax,* rodlet cells of the striped bass demonstrate no affinity for acid mucosubstances when stained by the alcian-blue–periodic-acid–Schiff technique. No inflammatory host response was associated with the rodlet cells examined in striped bass tissues. It is my opinion that these cells represent some stage in the life cycle of a sporazoan parasite.

Pseudobranchiae

The free pseudobranchiae of striped bass are located on the hyoid arch, occurring bilaterally along the inside of the opercula rostral to the first pair of gills (Fig. 19A). Although the pseudobranchiae resemble the gills both micro- and macroscopically, they receive oxygen-rich blood from the first efferent gill arteries and probably have no respiratory function in fish (Harder 1975). Within the pseudobranchiae, blood vessels split into a capillary system. Efferent arterial blood from these capillaries go to the choroid body of the eye, whereas venous blood is drained by the venous channels of the head, according to Parry and Holliday (1960).

Each pseudobranchia possesses a single row of filaments, unlike the paired hemobranchiae of the gill. Its epithelium is composed of acidophilic pseudobranchia cells and chloride cells, which are indistinguishable from one another by light microscopy in the striped bass (Fig. 19E). Mattey et al. (1978) indicated that, in the fish they examined, chloride cells of the pseudobranchiae contact the water directly by means of apical crypts, whereas the more abundant pseudobranchia cells are covered by a layer of squamous epithelium that isolates them from the environment. They also noted that pseudobranchia cells contain an orderly arrangement of parallel cytoplasmic tubules that are closely packed around abundant mitochondria. Conversely, the chloride cells contained irregularly arranged cytoplasmic tubules throughout the cytoplasm.

In both adult and age-0 striped bass, the pseudobranchia cells contain large apically placed nuclei (Fig. 19E). Rodlet cells and mucous cells are, however, more abundant in the epithelium of adult fish, whose secondary lamellae appear fused to one another by an outer epithelial layer. Cells occurring toward the bases of adjacent secondary lamellae often lack an overlying epithelium, suggesting the presence of distinct chloride cells in this region.

Copeland (1951) believed that the pseudobranchiae produce enzymes for use in the gas bladder. Parry and Holliday (1960) suggested several functions for this tissue: salt regulation; respiration; control of blood pressure to the eye or biochemical regulation of eye fluids; and production of hormones. They concluded that the pseudobranchia was involved in the maintenance of color in fish, by producing a chromatophore-concentrating hormone. Mattey et al. (1978) attribute enzymatic, endocrine, chemoreceptive, and osmoregulatory functions to this organ. To date, the question of function remains unresolved, although a large number of ionocytes within the pseudobranchia filaments supports a role in osmoregulation.

Renal Excretory System

The trunk kidney is one of the more important excretory organs of teleost fishes. Together with the skin, intestinal mucosa, liver, and gill epithelium, it maintains delicate osmotic balances between the fish and its environment. In euyhaline fish like the striped bass, the kidney must maintain this balance in both fresh and salt water. In fresh water, the trunk kidney and urinary bladder function in the excretion of a dilute urine, whereas in seawater, the same tissues must conserve water by producing a concentrated hypertonic urine. Because of this unique physiological trait, the striped bass trunk kidney has been the focus of several histomorphological studies (Beitch 1962, 1963; Bryant 1970; Bryant and Seibel 1970, 1971).

Bryant and Seibel (1970, 1971) investigated both pronephric and mesonephric tubulogenesis in larval striped bass. Their histological and ultrastructural findings were best summarized by Bryant (1970):

> The kidney of the striped bass . . . exhibits a transitional state between the evolutionary stages of glomerulization versus aglomerulization. In the freshwater environment, the glomerulated protion of the kidney is divisible into a nephron unit consisting of three histologically distinct segments, and a ureteric tree consisting of a tri-tubular branching system. The proximal nephron contains two distinct cell types, a "light" and a "dark" cell, exhibiting specific staining characteristics and differences in cytoplasmic inclusions. A third unusual cell form appears in the ureteric branches in addition to the typical cell types and contains hyalinized bodies enclosing specific inclusions (rodlet cells). During the larval development the newly hatched larvae possess an aglomerular pronephric kidney. Development of the mesonephric kidney appears during the early larval stages and is characterized by a decrease in salinity tolerance levels during the first week. . . . Subsequent maturation is characterized by gradual increase in salinity tolerances to forty-two parts per thousand by age twelve weeks. This value is higher than the average salinity of sea water. The presence of a mixed mesonephric kidney and the variation in salinity tolerance during development show a definite relationship to the variable environment of the striped bass during its life cycle.

Beitch (1962) noted that the trunk kidney of striped bass was located exterior to the dorsal wall of the peritoneal cavity and ventral to the axial skeleton (Fig. 1). The dense peritoneal connective tissue that covers the ventral surface of the trunk kidney forms a common wall with the gas bladder (Fig. 20 A,B). The left and right lobes of the hematopoietic head kidney are separated from each other, rostral to the fifth intervertebral segments (see Circulatory System, page 18). Conversely, the mesonephric lobes are united caudal to this segment. As with Kendall's and Hinton's (1974) findings for channel catfish, no renal cortex or medulla can be differentiated in this region. In addition, Beitch reported that the mean length of the mesonephros was approximately 30% of the standard length of the fish he examined. Harder (1975) classified this type of kidney, in which the entire mesonephros or opisthonephros is functional, as holotypic.

Beitch (1962) also reported that a ureter or opisthonephric duct is located on either side of the posterior trunk kidney (Fig. 20B). These ducts enter the posterior mesonephros, usually on the right side, and unite to form a single urinary duct caudal to the kidney. The renal portal veins (right and left caudal veins) enter the mesonephros laterally at a point rostral to that of the opistonephric ducts. The left branch of the caudal vein, medial

Figure 20. Trunk kidney of a 3-year-old striped bass.

- **A.** Sagittal section of trunk and head kidney tissue (formalin; H&E). Bar = 261 μm.
- **B.** Transverse section of the trunk kidney (formol sublimate; H&E). Bar = 332 μm.
- **C.** Trunk kidney (formalin; H&E). Bar = 43 μm.
- **D.** Oblique section through neck segment of a kidney tubule (formalin; H&E). Bar = 10.7 μm.
- **E.** Transverse section of first proximal kidney tubule segment (formalin; H&E). Bar = 7.8 μm.
- **F.** Transverse section of the second proximal kidney tubule segment (formalin; H&E). Bar = 7.5 μm.

1 Adipose tissue
2 Artery
3 Brush border (microvilli)
4 Collecting (opistonephric) duct
5 Collecting tubule
6 Cuboidal tubule cell
7 Distal tubule segment
8 Dorsal aorta
9 First proximal tubule segment
10 Glomerulus
11 Hematopoietic kidney tissue
12 Intercalated cell
13 Kidney tubules
14 Low columnar tubule cell
15 Lumen of the gas bladder
16 Posterior cardinal vein
17 Red blood cells
18 Reticular connective tissue
19 Second proximal tubule segment

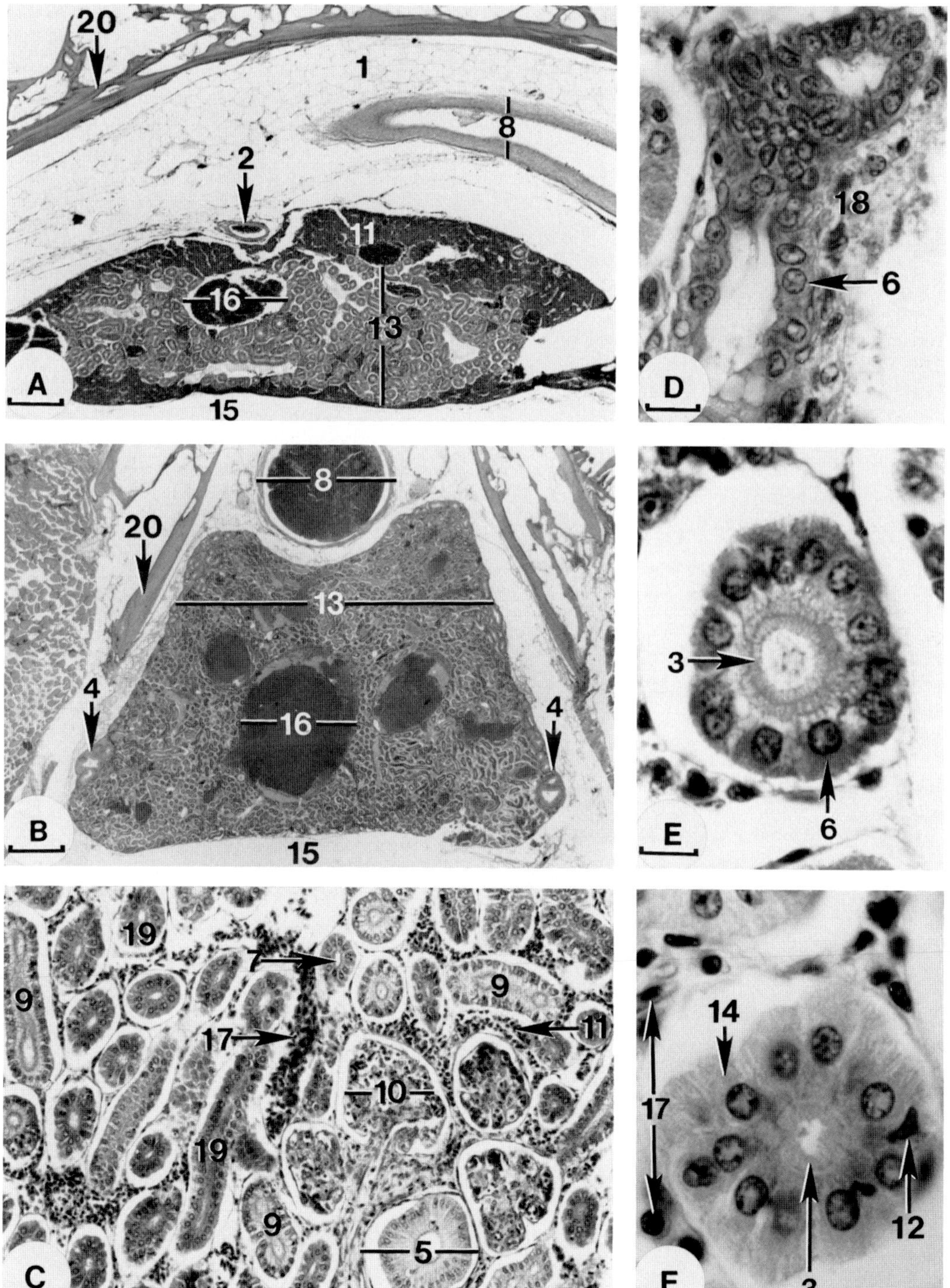
20
1
8
2
11
16
13
A
15
D
18
6
8
20
13
4
16
4
B
15
E
3
6
C
19
9
7
9
17
11
10
19
9
5
F
14
17
12
3

Figure 20

branches of the right posterior cardinal vein, and the segmental veins form the sinusoids of the trunk kidney. Blood sinusoids throughout the mesonephros are separated from the nephrons by a basement membrane and a thin reticular stroma. The venous channels, formed by the union of the blood sinusoids, enter the right posterior cardinal vein, which continues to the heart (Fig. 20A,B). This vein is very wide in the rostral mesonephros near the head kidney. According to Beitch (1962), blood sinusoids are lacking in the caudal trunk kidney of age-0 striped bass. Anderson and Anderson (1976) traced the renal vasculature of the rainbow and brook trout, and noted that the afferent blood originates from the dorsal aorta (Fig. 20A,B). Similarly, in striped bass, this aortic blood moves through the afferent glomerular arterioles into the glomerular tuft and exits via an efferent arteriole into the peritubular capillary beds and sinusoids. Blood from the sinusoids subsequently is collected within the caudal and posterior cardinal veins and returned to the heart.

Nephron

As noted above, the striped bass trunk kidney cannot be separated histologically into a renal medulla or cortex, unlike that of higher vertebrates. Rather, it is composed of identical nephrons that are the functional excretory units of the kidney (Fig. 20B,C). Each nephron contains a renal corpuscle and a renal tubule (Fig. 20D,E,F). The renal corpuscle contains a vascular capillary glomerulus that is enclosed by Bowman's capsule (Figs. 20C, 21A). This capsule contains an inner layer of visceral epithelium (podocytes) and an outer layer of parietal epithelium that separates the renal corpuscle from the rest of the kidney (Fig. 21A) (Patt and Patt 1969). According to Grizzle and Rogers (1976), the podocytes are separated from the endothelium by a basement membrane in channel catfish. The lumen formed between the two capsular epithelial wall is termed Bowman's space. Beitch (1962, 1963) found that the glomeruli and glomerular spaces were larger in striped bass examined from fresh water. This finding is in agreement with that of Olivereau and Olivereau (1977) for the European eel.

Blood flow to the glomerulus via the afferent glomerular arteriole is controlled partially by enzymatic secretions of the juxtaglomerular cells in fish as well as in higher vertebrates. These cells are located within the arteriole walls proximal to the glomerulus. The juxtaglomerular cells of teleosts develop out of smooth muscle cells and are considered the equivalents of those found in mammals (Harder 1975). They produce a proteolytic enzyme, renin, that is necessary for the production of angiotonin and the regulation of blood pressure. The striped bass juxtaglomerular cells are in direct contact with arteriole endothelium and often encircle the entire vessel. They appear hypertrophic, having a light, finely granular basophilic cytoplasm and a prominent, irregularly shaped nucleus that often conforms to the elongated shape of the cells. A histological confirmation of renin in striped bass was not part of this study although Oguri and Sokabe (1968) have stained this enzyme successfully in other teleosts.

The striped bass nephron has five tubular segments: neck; first proximal; second proximal; distal; and collecting. The neck segment is short and contains tightly packed basophilic cuboidal epi-

Figure 21. Trunk kidney and urinary bladder of a 3-year-old striped bass.

A. Renal corpuscle (glomerulus) (formalin; H&E). Bar = 20 μm.
B. Transverse section of a distal kidney tubule (left) and a collecting tubule (right) (formalin; H&E). Bar = 10 μm.
C. Transverse section of an opisthonephric duct in the trunk kidney (formol sublimate; H&E). Bar = 40 μm.
D. Urinary bladder epithelium (Bouin's; HPS). Bar = 18 μm.
E. Urinary bladder (Bouin's; HPS). Bar = 71 μm.

1 Adipose tissue
2 Artery
3 Bowman's space
4 Capillaries
5 Collecting ducts
6 Columnar epithelium
7 Dense connective tissue
8 Distal kidney tubule segment
9 Endothelial cell
10 Fibrous connective tissue and smooth muscle
11 Leukocytes
12 Low columnar tubule cell
13 Lumen of urinary bladder
14 Opisthonephric ducts
15 Parietal epithelium of renal capsule
16 Peripheral nerve
17 Pseudostratified columnar epithelium
18 Red blood cells
19 Reticular connective tissue
20 Rodlet cells
21 Second proximal kidney tubule segment
22 Smooth muscle fibers
23 Vein
24 Visceral epithelium of renal capsule (podocytes)
25 Wall of urinary bladder

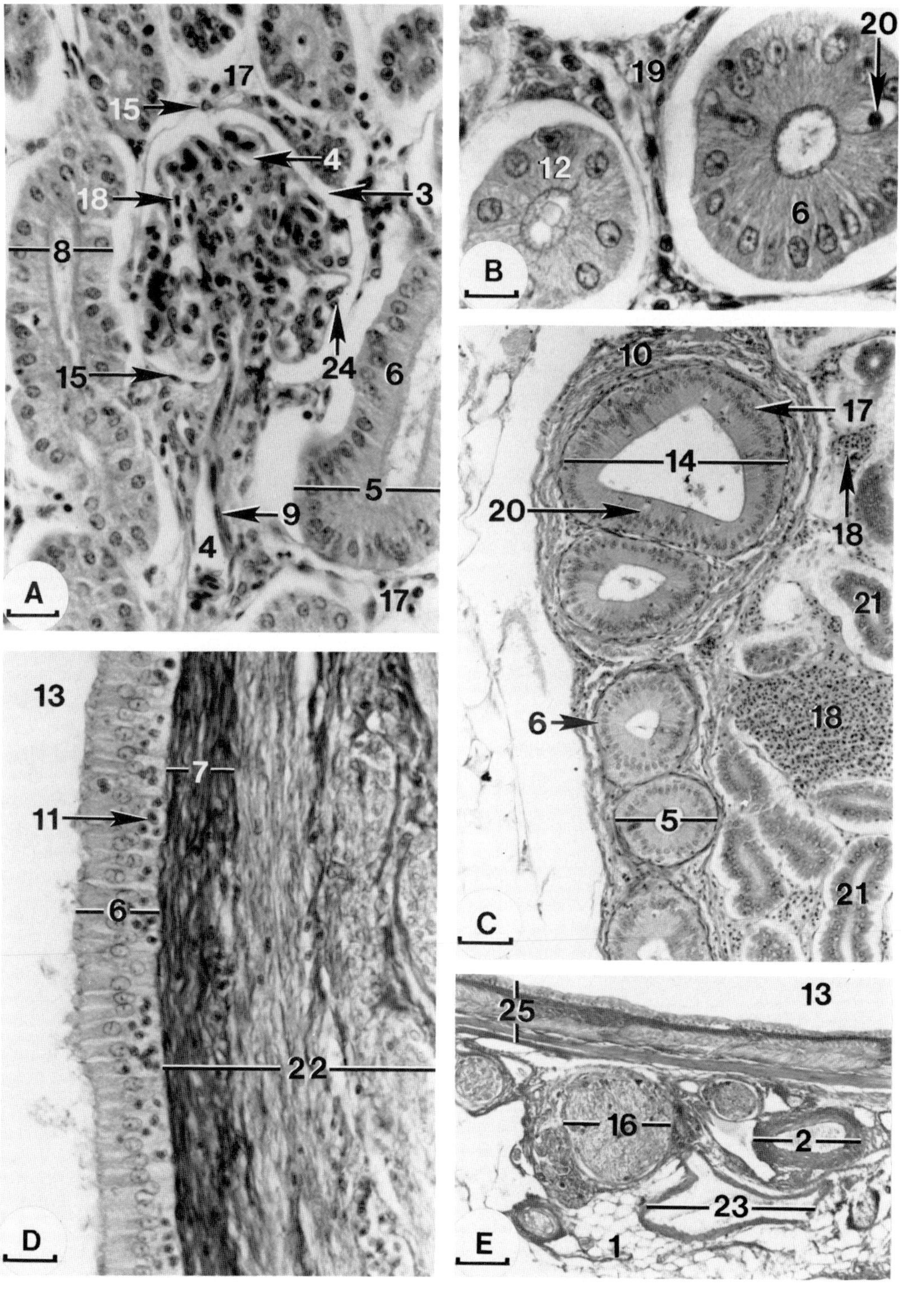
A
17
15
4
3
18
8
15
24
6
5
9
4
17
B
20
19
12
6
C
10
17
14
20
18
21
6
18
5
21
D
13
7
11
6
22
E
25
13
16
2
23
1

Figure 21

thelium (Fig. 20D) and is continuous with the parietal and visceral epithelium of Bowman's capsule. The centrally placed nucleus occupies more than one half of the cuboidal neck cell's cytoplasm. These tubular cells have no distinct brush border (microvilli) and most-nearly resemble those described by Olivereau and Olivereau (1977) for the European eel and Ottosen (1978) for the European plaice.

The first proximal segment begins with cuboidal, and ends in low columnar, epithelium that contains basally located, rounded nuclei (Fig. 20E). The supranuclear cytoplasm of each tubule cell stains less acidophilic than the basal cytoplasm. This suggests the presence of numerous endocytic vacuoles, lysosomes, and an extensive tubular system below a prominent brush border as has been reported also by Anderson and Mitchum (1974) for trout, and Ottosen (1978) for the European plaice. Both the tubular and lumen diameters are increased over those of the neck segment.

The columnar epithelium of the second proximal segment has a homogenous, strongly acidophilic-staining cytoplasm (Fig. 20F). These cells have central rounded nuclei, reduced brush borders, and narrower tubular lumens than those of the first proximal segment. Anderson and Mitchum (1974) suggested that this second segment may be responsible for divalent-ion secretion in teleosts. Intercalated cells (leukocytes) were evident here and throughout most of the renal tubules (Fig. 20F). They occurred between the tubular epithelial cells and generally contained irregular flattened nuclei and little surrounding cytoplasm (Grizzle and Rogers 1976).

No intermediate segment, as described by Kendall and Hinton (1974) for channel catfish, is found in the striped bass. However, a short distal segment is present (Fig. 21B). Cells of its low columnar epithelium have homogenous, slightly acidophilic cytoplasm and basally located nuclei, but lack a brush border. According to Anderson and Mitchum (1974) and Hentschel (1978), this segment functions in the conservation of salts and, consequently, is reduced or nonfunctional in marine teleosts. Beitch (1962) noted that a distal segment was absent in the striped bass he examined from seawater. The length and number of classical distal tubules found in striped bass are less than have been reported for trout (Anderson and Mitchum 1974). Consequently, collecting tubules comprised a greater percentage of the fourth nephron segment. They are distinguished from the distal tubules by an increase in tubular cell size (cuboidal to tall columnar), cell number, lumen and tubular dimeters, cellular basophilia, and the addition of an external connective tissue layer (Figs. 20C, 21B,C). This fibrous connective tissue appears in the larger collecting tubules that are located proximal to the major opisthonephric ducts (Fig. 21C). Rodlet cells are increasingly evident in this segment of the renal tubules (Fig. 21B). In contrast to the report by Beitch (1962), no goblet cells were found in any of the bass collecting tubules examined in this study.

Opisthonephric Ducts and Urinary Bladder

The two lateral opisthonephric ducts connect the nephron with the urinary duct and transport urine to the urinary bladder. The duct wall contains a pseudostratified columnar epithelium whose cells resemble those of the larger collecting ducts. Smooth muscle fibers are present between the lumen epithelium and the outer fibrous connective tissue layer. The walls of the opisthonephric ducts enlarge as they unite to form the urinary duct. A distinct serosa surrounds the peritoneal surfaces of the urinary duct and the urinary bladder of striped bass. This serosa contains an outer mesothelial layer and a thin layer of underlying connective tissue, similar to that in channel catfish (Grizzle and Rogers 1976).

The urinary bladder is located along the caudal wall of the peritoneal cavity (Fig. 1). Its dorsocaudal wall is fused to the body musculature and its ventrorostral wall borders the peritoneal cavity. Because it originates from the urinary and opisthonephric ducts, it is considered a morphological and functional extension of the trunk kidney (Howe and Gutknecht 1978). When the bladder is distended, its epithelium appears cuboidal; when it is empty, these same cells can appear columnar (Fig. 21D). Each cell has a homogenous, slightly acidophilic cytoplasm and a central or basally situated, oval nucleus. Leukocytes and rodlet cells are especially prominent directly under the epithelium, which is surrounded externally by smooth muscle bundles. Peripheral nerve bundles, blood vessels, and loose connective tissue are present both under the serosal surface and proximal to the body wall that abutts the urinary bladder. As reported by Nagahama et al. (1975) for the longjaw mudsucker, no mucous cells were present in the epithelium of the striped bass examined. The urinary bladder narrows ventrally to form a channel or urinary pore that exits the body caudal to both the anus and genital pore. In some marine teleosts, the urinary bladder can resorb water and sodium, chloride, magnesium, and sulphate ions (Howe and Gutknect 1978).

Reproductive System

Striped bass are oviparous, although about 3% are hermaphroditic according to Dorfman (1976). Among females, 25% spawn after 4 years, 75% after 5 years, and 95% after 6 years, whereas most males spawn at age 2. Both sexes can spawn in successive years. The fecundity of a 4.5-year-old female ranges between 200,000 and 700,000 eggs. Spawning of anadromous stocks occurs in brackish estuaries or in turbulent areas of freshwater rivers. Where striped bass occur as landlocked populations, they may spawn in actively moving tributary waters of lakes and reservoirs. The spawning season extends from April to July, but varies with water temperature and latitude (Table 1).

Striped bass normally possess paired elongated testes or ovaries along the dorsal wall of the body cavity. The testes produce motile sperm and the ovaries pelagic eggs. These organs are suspended directly from the ventral surface of the gas bladder by short peritoneal mesenteries (Harder 1975); these mesenteries are continuations of the parietal peritoneum that extends from either side of the gas bladder and trunk kidney. This peritoneum continues laterally around, and attaches to, the ventral surface of each gonad (Cooper 1952). Gonadal arteries, veins, lymphatic ducts, and nerves enter each gonad via the rostral mesenteric attachments and branch profusely as they continue caudally along the mid-dorsal wall within the tunica albuginea (Fig. 22A). The tunica albuginea comprises the peripheral wall of the gonad and is continuous with the thinner interstitial or capsular walls of the seminiferous tubules and ovigerous lamellae (Anderson and Mitchum 1974; Grizzle and Rogers 1976). The gonads unite caudally to form a common genital duct that exits the body through the genital orifice, between the anus and the urinary pore (Harder 1975). The tissue immediately dorsal to the wall of the pore is densely supplied with heavy bands of elastic fibers, areolar connective tissue, bundles of striated muscle fibers, and dense areas of adipose tissue. In addition to gamete production, the teleost gonads also produce hormones as noted by Grizzle and Rogers (1976).

Ovary

The striped bass ovary has two lobes that join caudally, forming a single bilobed organ with a short oviduct that exits between the anus and the urinary pore. The oviduct is lined by a thick squamous epithelium and surrounded by dense connective tissue. The mesenteries that suspend the ovarian lobes from the ventral surface of the gas bladder are termed mesovaria (Harder 1975). The major blood vessels, lymphatic ducts, and nerves that supply the ovary enter via this tissue. In striped bass, as in largemouth bass and bluegills (James 1946), the mesovaria are continuous with peritoneal or thick mesothelial covering of the ovarian wall, or tunica albuginea (Fig. 22A,B). Within the fibrous connective tissue of the tunica albuginea are anastomosing circular and longitudinal smooth muscle bundles that are heavily invaded with collagen (Fig 22B). Branches of the gonadal blood vessels, lymphatic ducts, and nerves run throughout this wall. The lumenal border of the ovarian wall is a thick squamous epithelium continuous with the lumenal surface epithelium of the ovigerous lamellae (Fig. 22A,C). These lamellar projections are perpendicular to the long axis of each ovarian lobe. The thin lamellar wall contains germinal epithelium, follicular epithelium, blood vessels, and a connective tissue stroma (Fig. 22C,D). The walls branch profusely within the lamellar lumen to form dendritic patterns of fibrovascular stromata, the surface of which is covered with oocytes at various stages of maturation; Moser (1967) described a similar pattern for the boccacio.

Oogenesis in the striped bass occurs within the ovigerous lamellae. It begins with mitosis of primary germ cells or oogonia that subsequently undergo meiosis to form oocytes. Oogonia are released from the germinal epithelium of the lamellae and mature within the dendritic folds of follicular epithelium (Harder 1975; Grizzle and Rogers 1976). Harder (1975), in a discussion of oogenesis, noted that after meiosis begins, one of the daughter oogonia contains a disproportionately large amount of oviplasm and develops into a secondary oocyte. This oocyte remains in the prophase of meiosis, during which time the oviplasm increases and the follicle develops.

Six oocytic maturation stages occur in the mature striped bass ovary prior to spawning. These stages are similar to those described for Gulf menhaden by Combs (1969). Juvenile females are easily identified histologically by the presence of numerous immature ova (stages I, II, and III) within the ovigerous lamellae (Merriman 1941). A mature female contains oogonia and oocytes in several stages of maturation prior to spawning. Merriman (1941) noted that oocytes developed more uniformly throughout the ovary as spring approached. Stage-I ova are undifferentiated oogonia that develop out of the germinal epithelium of the lamellar stroma (Fig. 22D). These cells occur in nests and contain lightly acidophilic-staining cytoplasm with large rounded central nuclei each containing a prominent nucleolus. Stage-II ova are larger and stain basophilically; each contains a disproportionately large central nucleus with diffuse chromatin (Fig. 22D). These primary oocytes represent the initial stage (prophase) of meiosis (Harder 1975). As primary oocytes mature, they become enveloped by a follicular epithelium, develop eccentrically located nucleoli, and move away from the lamellar wall. Combs (1969) noted that primary oocytes may be present in the ovary throughout the year in Gulf menhaden. I also found this to be true for striped bass. Wallace and Selman (1981) refer to this as the primary growth stage or chromatin nucleolar stage in oocyte maturation.

Hurley and Fisher (1966), in a discussion of the follicle of the oviparous teleost egg, noted that the vitelline membrane forms the boundary of the oviplasm. This membrane also surrounds the microvilli that pass through the pore canals of the zona radiata and project into the clear homogenous zona pellucida or chorion of the ovum. The fluid absorbed by the egg during the water-hardening process accumulates between the vitelline membrane and the zona radiata, which hardens after fertilization. The micropyle is located in the zona radiata, which also contains microvilli that histologically appear as striations. Harder (1975) noted that the microvilli help in the pinocytosis of vitellogenin by the maturing ovum. Follicular cells that encircle a stage-II oocyte form a single layer in striped bass, like those of medaka (Tesoriero 1977). According to Hurley and Fisher (1966), teleost follicular cells are enclosed by the membrana propria folliculi, which consists of a laminated series of membranes and a thin thecal cell layer containing the blood vessel of the follicle. In the striped bass, no zona pellucida or thecal cell layer is evident by light microscopy, although they may be present.

Stage-III ova of the striped bass are large oocytes that have a well-developed follicular epithelium (Fig. 22B,C,D,E) and a dramatically increased basophilic oviplasm in comparison to stage-II ova. Wallace and Selman (1981) noted that perinuclear basophilic accumulation during growth "nuage" is comprised of ribonucleic protein particles. The nucleus stains acidophilically, and numerous provitelline nucleoli appear in the karyoplasm as the true nucleolus migrates to a more peripheral position. Migration of the provitelline nucleoli toward the nuclear membrane results in the formation of euvitelline nucleoli that are believed to be involved with ribonucleic acid synthesis. This process coincides with lipogenesis in teleosts and has been termed the perinucleolar stage.

In stage-IV ova, the oviplasm begins to stain basophilically, euvitelline nucleoli appear along the nuclear membrane, the nucleus stains acidophilically, and no true nucleolus is evident. This stage signals the beginning of yolk-vesicle formation and vitellogenesis (Wallace and Selman 1981). An increase in yolk granules and fat vacuoles occurs in the oviplasm and a distinct zona radiata can be distinguished in the follicular epithelium for the first time. In stage-V ova, there is a tremendous increase in yolk vesicles, except in the basophillic blue-grey oviplasm directly adjacent to the acidophilic nucleus (Fig. 22E). Similarly, a thin

Figure 22. Female reproductive system of striped bass.

A. Transverse section of a juvenile ovary (formalin; H&E). Bar = 267 μm.
B. Wall of the ovary proximal to the oviduct, juvenile fish (formalin; H&E). Bar = 71 μm.
C. Primary follicles (stages I, II, III) within the ovigenous lamellae, juvenile fish (formol sublimate; H&E). Bar = 43 μm.
D. Nests of oogonia in a juvenile ovary, juvenile fish (Bouin's; H&E). Bar = 43 μm.
E. Maturing oocytes stage V (center) and stage VI (bottom left), 3-year-old fish (formalin; H&E). Bar = 24 μm.

1 Cytoplasm of oocyte stage V
2 Euvitelline nucleoli
3 Fibrous connective tissue stroma
4 Follicular cells
5 Lumen of ovary
6 Nucleus of oocyte (karyoplasm and provitelline nucleoli)
7 Oocyte stage I (oogonial nest)
8 Oocyte stage II
9 Oocyte stage III
10 Ovarian vein
11 Ovigerous lamellae with immature oocytes
12 Provitelline nucleoli
13 Red blood cell
14 Smooth muscle bundles
15 Tunica albuginea
16 Yolk granules
17 Yolk vacuoles

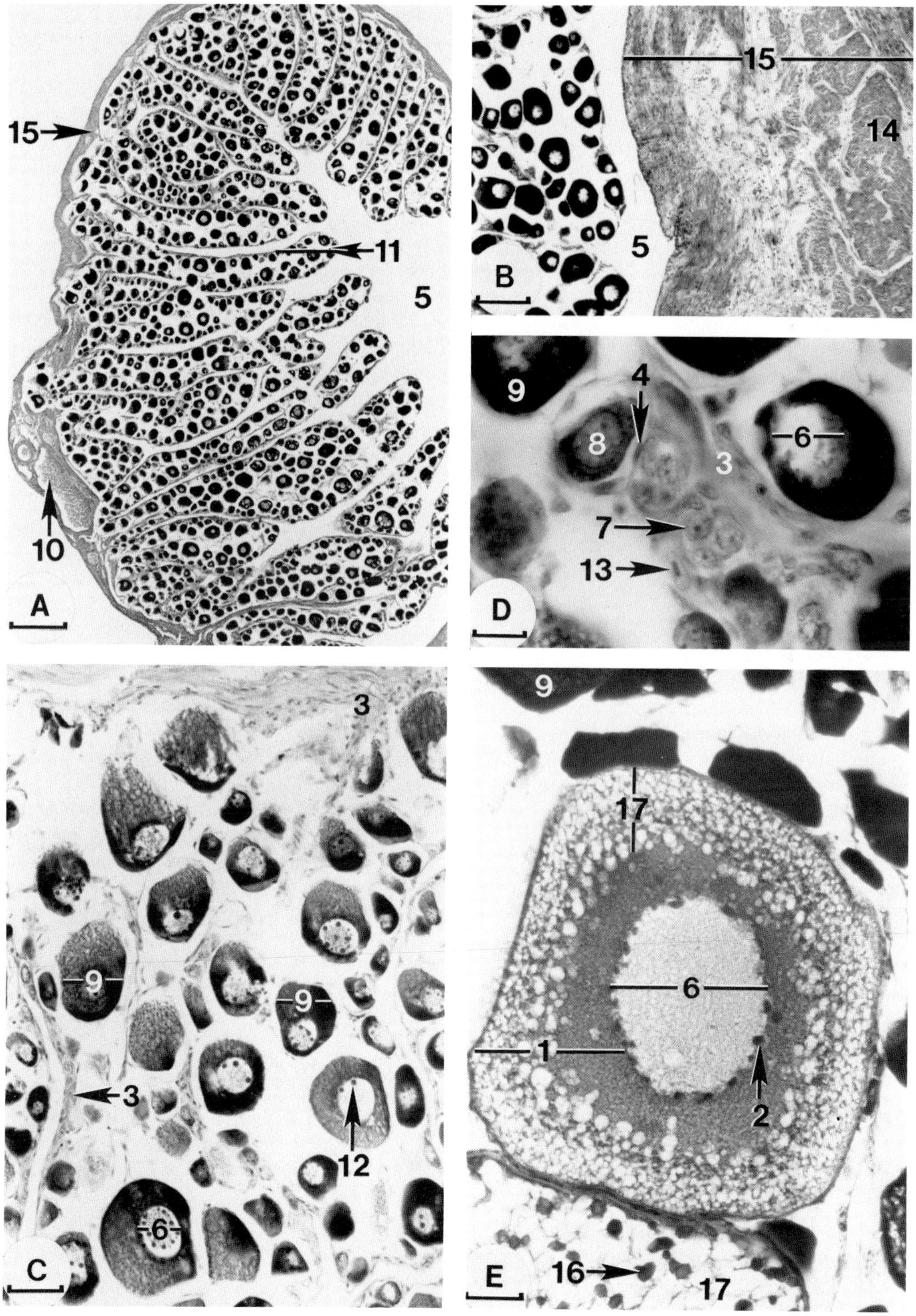

Figure 22

ring of unvacuolated blue-grey oviplasm is located beneath the zona radiata and fewer euvitelline nucleoli are present in the acidophilic nucleus. At this stage, both the nuclear membrane and karyoplasm are degenerating. Stage-VI ova contain oviplasm filled with larger fat vacuoles and acidophilic yolk granules, except for a thin layer of homogenous blue-grey cytoplasm that remains adjacent to the zona radiata (Fig. 22E).

In many teleosts, the conclusion of maturation is thought to be preceded by the migration of the nucleus or germinal vesicle of a stage-VI ovum to a peripheral position near the zona radiata and micropyle, where the initial meiosis is completed and the first polar body is formed. Subsequently, a second meiosis occurs, producing three haploid bodies that all eventually degenerate, and a large haploid ovum that develops into a mature egg (Wallace and Selman 1981).

With pelagic eggs, like those of striped bass, the large fat vacuoles function as flotation devices following release of the eggs from the female. Mature eggs range in diameter from 1.0 to 1.35 mm when deposited (Westin and Rogers 1978) and take 30–74 hours to hatch, depending upon water temperature (Table 1).

Hoar (1965) stated that there was no general agreement on the locus of hormone production in the ovary of fish, but suggested that some teleost yolk has a high estrogen content. Grizzle and Rogers (1976) suggested that both estrogen and progesterone are produced by the ovarian follicle or corpus lutea (atretic follicle), but this has not been confirmed. The ovaries examined in this study did not contain atretic follicles and no special stains were employed to detect cells that produce estrogen or progesterone. Interstitial tissue, containing tissue macrophages and epithelial elements that may represent endocrine tissue, was noted between developing oocytes.

Testis

Striped bass, like largemouth bass and bluegills (James 1946), have bilobed testes that are attached to the gas bladder by mesenteries termed mesorchia (Fig. 23A). Each testicular lobe forms a radial testis that contains a regular system of lobules or seminiferous tubules (Harder 1975). These tubules radiate perpendicularly from a central longitudinal collecting duct (ductus deferens) and terminate blindly at the periphery of the lobe beneath the thin tunica albuginea (Fig. 23B) like those of the bocaccio (Moser 1967). A thick squamous peritoneal mesothelium (mesorchia) covers the thin tunica albuginea, which contains fibrous connective tissue, melanocytes, smooth muscle cells, collagen fibers, gonadal arteries, veins, and peripheral nerves. (According to Grier 1981, teleost testes lack of lymphatic system. This was not confirmed for the striped bass.) This outer wall penetrates the testis to form thin capsules around each seminiferous tubule (Fig. 23C) (Moser 1967). The tubules connect with the ductus deferens toward the center of each lobe. The wall of the ductus deferens consists of both smooth muscle fibers and fibrous connective tissue. It is lined by a low cuboidal epithelium that contains scattered mucous cells at its junction with the seminiferous tubules. The two ductus deferens merge caudally and exit through the genital orifice, as noted above (Harder 1975).

Spermatogenesis in the striped bass occurs along the entire length of the tubules. Grier (1981) classified this as an unrestricted spermatogonial testis. Juvenile males lack a well-defined tubular system, but have numerous primordial germ-cell cysts (Fig. 23D). The germ cells, or primary spermatogonia, resemble those described by Drance et al. (1976) for rainbow trout as being large, spherical, and acidophillic with moderately dense chromatin and a single prominent nucleolus in each.

Figure 23. Male reproductive system of striped bass.

A. Transverse section of an immature testis, 3-month-old fish (formalin; H&E). Bar = 259 μm.
B. Oblique section through the radial testis, 3-year-old fish; fixed during February (Bouin's; H&E). Bar = 81 μm.
C. Transverse section of the seminiferous tubule, 3-year-old fish, fixed during February (Bouin's; H&E). Bar = 17 μm.
D. Germinal cells of the testis, 3-month-old fish (formalin; H&E). Bar = 9.5 μm.
E. Mature spermatozoa, 3-year-old fish (Bouin's; H&E). Bar = 10 μm.

1 Collecting duct (ductus deferens)
2 Fibrous connective tissue of the Tunical albuginea
3 Gas-bladder wall
4 Genital artery
5 Genital vein
6 Head of spermatozoa
7 Interstitial cells
8 Mesenteric attachment (mesorchia)
9 Nest of primary spermatocytes
10 Nest of secondary spermatocytes
11 Primary spermatogonia
12 Secondary spermatogonia
13 Seminiferous tubule (lobule)
14 Spermatids
15 Spermatozoa
16 Tail of spermatozoa

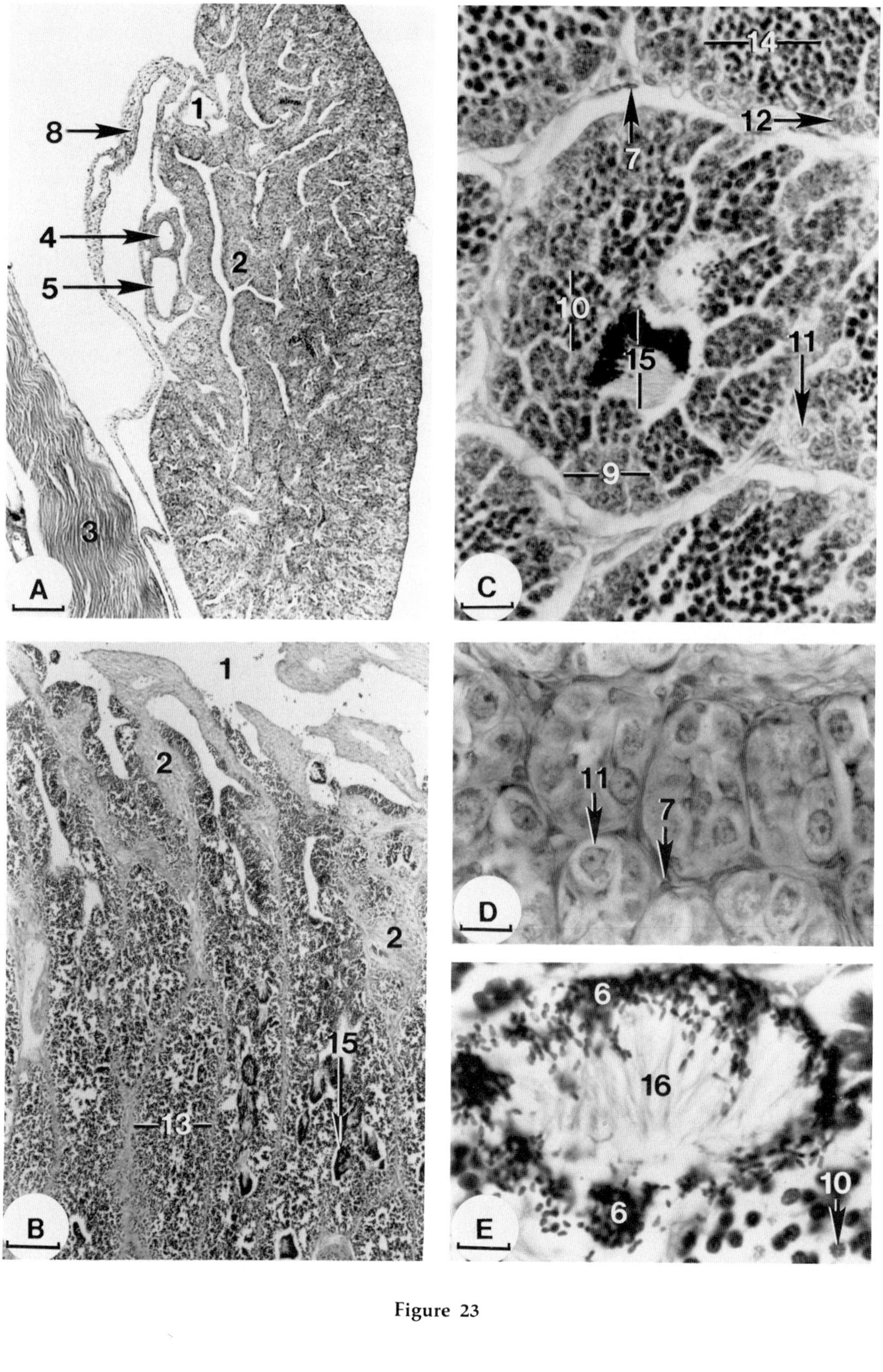

Figure 23

Generally, five to seven of these cells are present in a transverse section of the primordial tubules. Tubules of juvenile fish are encircled by thin flattened interstitial cells that comprise the fibrous capsule of the mature seminiferous tubules. Often the Sertoli cells or lobular boundary cells cannot be differentiated at this early stage of testicular development. In both juvenile and adult striped bass, primary spermatogonia migrate inward from germinal epithelium of the fibrous capsule and lodge among the Sertoli cells of the seminiferous tubules. There they later divide into secondary spermatogonia that resemble those described by Moser (1967) for the bocaccio.

In sexually mature male fish, six cellular stages can be differentiated in sperm maturation: primary and secondary spermatogonia; primary and secondary spermatocytes; spermatids; and spermatozoa (Fig. 23C). Striped bass produce sperm on a yearly cycle. Mature males, however, may contain several or all of the above cellular stages simultaneously prior to spawning. During spawning, the seminiferous tubules are filled primarily with mature spermatozoa (Fig. 23E). At the periphery of each tubule, enclosed within the fibers of connective tissue, are primary spermatogonia. Within the lumenal margins of the seminiferous tubules are cyst-like structures, each containing sperm cells of similar maturity. These cysts are enclosed by a single-cell-layered capsule that originates from the wall of the tubule just as in white and black crappies (Cooper 1952). According to Grier (1981), these cysts are formed by Sertoli cells in all teleost testes. In general, cysts containing more mature stages of sperm cells are located toward the inside of the tubule (Fig. 23C).

From each of the primary spermatogonia, a cyst is formed. Following a series of mitoses the cyst becomes filled with secondary spermatogonia (James 1946). A second series of mitotic divisions results in the formation of a cyst full of primary spermatocytes that have more condensed nuclei than the spermatogonia and stain basophilically. For most teleost fishes, the first meiotic division results in the formation of secondary spermatocytes, which still are held within the cysts. Secondary spermatocytes are smaller than primary ones, and have distinct cell membranes, large nuclei, reduced cytoplasm, scattered darkly staining chromatin, and no visible nucleoli (Harder 1975). These cells eventually burst the cyst capsule and are liberated into the tubular lumen where they complete maturation to become spermatids (Cooper 1952). A second meiosis is required to produce the spermatids. Each spermatid develops into a spermatozoan. A spermatid has a condensed, intensely basophilic-staining nucleus with chromatin that collects to one side in the advanced stages of maturation. Mature spermatozoa possess a distinct rounded basophilic head and a long acidophilic tail or flagellum (Fig. 23E); they congregate in the lumen of the tubule with tails close together and heads fanning out, resembling the shape of an umbrella (James 1946).

Neither Sertoli cells nor Leydig cells were histochemically identified in striped bass testes; however, Grier (1981) noted that both cell types are common to all teleosts. Similarly, Patt and Patt (1969) indicated that Sertoli cells are present in all vertebrate testes and function as nurse cells by holding spermatogenic cells within tubular cysts until spermatogenesis is completed. Drance et al. (1976) found that in rainbow trout, Sertoli cells can be identified by their angular contour and irregularly shaped nucleus. No cells fitting these descriptions were observed in the testes examined in this study; however, this does not preclude their existence. Although Marshall and Lofts (1956) described two types of Leydig cell homologues in teleosts (an interstitial gland composed of aggregations of modified connective-tissue cells and an intralobular gland that occur within the tubule wall), Grier (1981) indicated that only the interstitium of the testes contains these cells. Leydig cells secrete androgens that aid in the development of secondary sexual characteristics and the release of sperm from the tubules at spawning. Hoar (1965) further noted that intracellular androgens are produced in large quantities just prior to spawning and can be most readily identified with the aid of differential sudanophilic and cholesterol-positive stains. Grier (1981), however, explained that certain species of fish lack lipophilic material in their Leydig cells and suggested that lipophilia not be the only criterion explored when Leydig homology is determined.

The striped bass testes examined during this study were obtained from males prior to the onset of spawning and they appeared to lack distinct Leydig homologues. However, because no special histochemical or ultrastructural techniques were employed to identify androgen-producing cells, they may have been present. Vacuolated tissue macrophages and coarse eosinophillic granular leukocytes were noted within the intertubular connective tissue and tunica albuginea of the striped bass testes.

Integumentary System

The integument of the striped bass includes the skin, scales, and fins, and covers the entire body of the fish. The thickness of the skin varies in different regions of the body, being greatest in areas such as the head with large dermal and hypodermal layers (Anderson and Mitchum 1974; Grizzle and Rogers 1976). The skin functions in immunosurveillance and transports or excludes various environmental substances (Whitear 1977). In particular, it acts as a barrier to microorganisms, resists mechanical damage from various abrasions or shocks, and serves in the exchange of gases, water, ions, and larger molecules (respiration and osmoregulation). It also has a variety of secretory (mucoid and cuticular) and sensory (chemo- and neurosensory) functions (Leonard and Summers 1976). The scales lend both structural rigidity and protection to the integument, and the fins function primarily in spatial orientation, stabilization, and propulsion.

Skin

The skin consists of an epidermis, a dermis, and, in some regions of the integument, a hypodermis (Harder 1975). The striped bass epidermis is composed of a living stratified squamous epithelium in three layers: stratum basale or germinativum; fusiform layer; and mucous coat or cuticular layer. In adult fish, the thickness of the epidermis can range from a few cells along the lining of the nasal pits (Fig. 24A) to 10 or 20 cells above the scales proximal to the vent (Fig. 24B). The stratum basale is a single layer of columnar epithelium. It is situated on a thin basement membrane that can only be identified by histochemical staining or electron microscopy. These epithelial cells often appear distorted (conical or club-shaped) due to the presence of numerous leukocytes (Fig. 24C). The epidermal nuclei of the stratum basale are larger, less dense, and more uniformly ovoid than those of the remaining epidermal layers. Conversely, the nuclei of the cells in the fusiform layer appear dense and irregularly shaped (Anderson and Mitchum 1974; Burton 1978). These cells possess rigid peripheral walls composed of tonofibrils, according to Leonard and Summers (1976). In addition to the epithelial cells, mucous cells, tastebuds, and neuromasts may be located within the epidermis (see Sensory System, page 82). Epidermal cells appear cuboidal in the proximal region of the fusiform layer and squamous along its surface or distal region. Hunter and Nayudu (1978) noted that specific fingerprint-like surface patterns or whorl arrangements of microfolds are present on the surface of the teleost epidermis. These patterns generally are most prominent above scales and are lacking from the gill and corneal surfaces. The presence of such ridges was not investigated in striped bass.

In all teleosts, a cuticular layer of mucus covers the squamous epithelium, and is derived from the mucus cells located throughout the epidermis. In the striped bass, mucus cells occur both in the stratum basale and the epidermal surface. They contain flat basally located nuclei similar to Type-A mucus cells of the oral cavity, and are filled with glycoproteins. When stained by the alcian-blue–periodic-acid–Schiff technique, they are positive for sialomucins and sulphomucins. Gona (1979) noted that the sulphate glycoproteins may aid in combatting bacterial and fungal infections. No distinct cuticle and few mucus cells were present in the fish I examined; however, Roberts (1978) found that cuticular elements may be removed during routine tissue-processing for histology. When present, the teleost cuticle is the first barrier between the fish and the environment; it protects the epidermis, decreases the danger of wounding, prevents water penetration by osmosis, and reduces friction during swimming (Harder 1975).

The dermis serves as a tissue connection between the epidermis and the underlying dermal skeleton or musculature. In juvenile striped bass, the dermis is only a narrow stratum compactum composed of dense collagen fibers, elastic fibers, melanocytes, and few connective tissue cells (Figs. 24C–E, 33C–E). In adult fish, the dermis consists of an outer papillary layer (stratum compactum), which contains the dense collagen fibers, and an inner stratum spongiosa of loose connective tissue. This inner portion contains many cell types (coarse eosinophilic granular leukocytes, leukocytes, nerve cells, pigment cells), lymphatic ducts, and blood vessels that nourish the skin (Fig. 24A) (Harder 1975). The stratum spongiosa generally is widest in the integument of the head (Grizzle and Rogers 1976), although in striped bass it also makes up most of the dermis surrounding the scale pockets. No epidermal melanophores were noted; however, superficial dermal melanophores are present in two bands, one between the epidermis and the papillary layer and the other between the papillary layer and the stratum spongiosa (Fig. 24C,E) (Burton 1978). In addition to melanin, fish pigment cells can contain carotenoids, pterin, guanine crystals, or related pigments (Junqueira et al. 1978). Harder (1975) noted that quanine crystals contribute structural coloration by refecting light, thus emparting a silvery color to many fishes, including striped bass.

The hypodermis is between the stratum spongiosa and the underlying skeletal or muscular elements. It is composed primarily of areolar connective tissue and occurs mainly along the flanks of the fish, where it also binds the red and white myomeres to the integument. The hypodermis and stratum spongiosa are indistinguishable from one another in some regions of the integument, such as the head (Fig. 24E).

Scales

Harder (1975) noted that teleost scales are acellular dermal bone composed of a mineralized isopedine matrix enclosing thick orthogonally arranged collagen fibers. They are anchored within the dermal scale pockets that lie between layers of collagen fibers in the stratum spongiosa and the basement membrane of the epidermis (Fig. 24B). Portions of the upper and lower surfaces of each scale are covered by epidermis. Three types of cells are associated with scales in teleosts: hyposquamal; episquamal; and peripheral (Harder 1975). Flat hyposquamal cells occur as two or three layers directly beneath the fibrous layer of the scale and are attached to one another at their edges. Episquamal cells cover the anterior and lateral fields on the external side of the scale. Scale radii are formed by peripheral radius cells that penetrate vertically through the scale and connect the hypo- and episquamal cells. The striped bass has ctenoid scales that are histologically similar to the above description. They are arranged in an overlapping pattern with their free edges directed caudad covering all of the body except the head and fins. Scales can be regenerated.

Fins

Teleost fins are broad-surfaced folds of skin that can contain special support elements: soft fin rays and hard spines. All fins are integrated with the skeletal muscular system through these support elements. The soft segmented rays contain paired lepidotrichia that are divided lengthwise, each being separated and arranged in a bilaterally symmetrical fashion, whereas the hard unsegmented rays or spines occur singularly (Harder 1975; Grizzle and Rogers 1976). The lepidotrichia develop from scales and similarly are composed of dermal bone (Fig. 24D). Each pair of lepidotrichia like those of the striped bass are considered phylogenetically recent.

The striped bass has unpaired dorsal, anal, and caudal fins, along with paired pelvic and pectoral fins (Figs. 1 and 2). The dorsal and anal fins contain both soft fin rays and hard spines (Manseuti 1958) (Figs. 1, 25C, 26C). Each fin is covered by a stratified squamous epithelium that is continuous with the epidermis of the fish. With the exception of a reduced stratum compactum and an increased hypodermis, the skin overlying the fins is indistinguishable from that found in the rest of the striped bass integument.

Figure 24. Integumentary system of striped bass.

A. Integument of the nasal cavity, 3-year-old fish (formol sublimate; H&E). Bar = 43 μm.
B. Overlapping scales of the ventral integument, 3-year-old fish (formalin; H&E). Bar = 44 μm.
C. Epidermis and dermis of the head, 3-year-old fish (formol sublimate; H&E). Bar = 16 μm.
D. Transverse section of a pelvic fin, 3-month-old fish (formalin; H&E). Bar = 69 μm.
E. Integument of the head, 3-year-old fish (formol sublimate; H&E). Bar = 59 μm.

1 Areolar connective tissue
2 Chromatophores (melanocytes)
3 Dermis (stratum compactum)
4 Fusiform layer
5 Hypodermis and stratum spongiosa
6 Lepidotrichia
7 Lumen of the nasal cavity
8 Papillary layer of the dermis
9 Peripheral nerve
10 Scale (dermal bone)
11 Scale pocket
12 Stratified squamous epithelium
13 Statum germinativum (stratum basale)
14 Venule
15 Wandering leukocytes

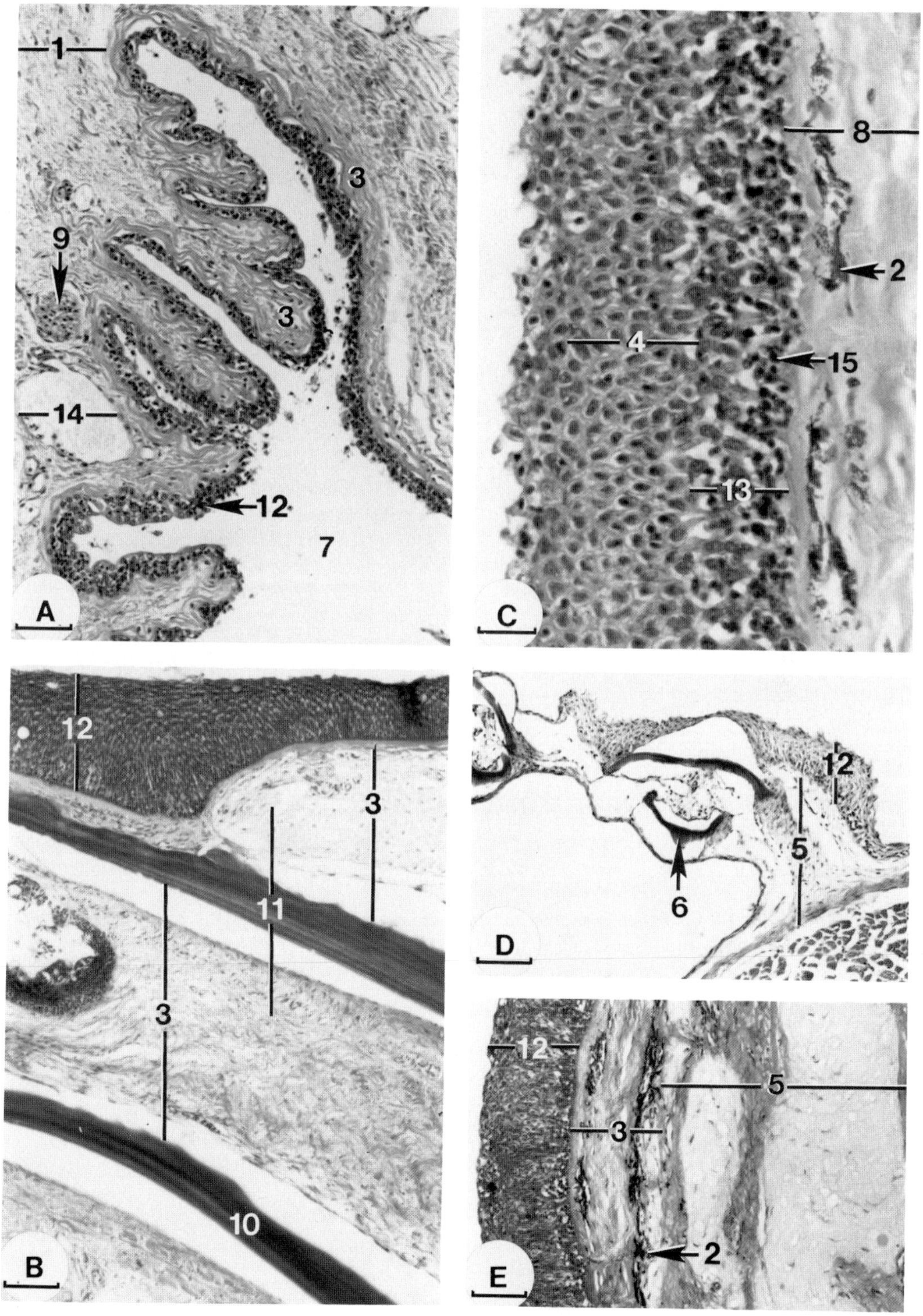

Figure 24

Muscular System

The muscular system constitutes the largest portion of the teleost body. It functions in overall body locomotion, coordinated movement of skeletal elements, pumping of blood, and peristaltic constrictions of visceral organs and their related structures (Grizzle and Rogers 1976). Cells and fibers of vertebrate muscle contain contractile myofibrils, noncontractile sarcoplasm, and membranes or sarcolemma that send deep invaginations into the sarcoplasm; these invaginations comprise the T-system (tubuli system) (Harder 1975). Three types of muscle tissue occur in teleosts: skeletal; smooth; and cardiac. Smooth muscle is composed of mononuclear muscle cells, whereas the other two contain multinucleated muscle fibers that are joined by facia of connective tissue (endomysium) to form muscle bundles.

Skeletal, or striated, muscle is found exclusively in tissues subject to voluntary control. Its multinucleate fibers contain myofibrils that are spread evenly over the entire cross section, concentrated around the center, or located along the fiber wall (Harder 1975). The myofibrils are composed of hundreds of myofilaments divided into thin (actin) and thick (myosin) elements. In combination, these filaments form regular striated patterns that have been designated as specific zones or bands. The A-bands contain myosin filaments and the I-bands contain actin filaments (Fig. 25A). Oval nuclei are located peripherally beneath the sarcolemma of each muscle fiber (Fig. 25A,B). These nuclei should not be confused with the more condensed nuclei of the endomysial cells that join muscle fibers into bundles. According to Harder (1975), the T-system noted above transmits action potentials from the sarcolemma to the proximity of the fiber bundles.

Locomotion of striped bass occurs principally by alternate contractions of muscles on each side of the body. These skeletal muscles, necessary for quick powerful contractions, are composed chiefly of segmental myomeres, the number of which correspond with that of the vertebrae: 24 in striped bass (Fig. 2). Each myomere is regarded as a separate muscle and its fibers are parallel to the long axis of the body (Fig. 25C,D). These fibers insert into broad sheets of collagenous connective tissue termed myosepta, which are attached to the vertebrae (Harder 1975; Grizzle and Rogers 1976). The epaxial myomeres are located along the dorsolateral body wall (Fig. 25C), whereas the hypaxial myomeres form the ventrolateral body wall (see page 65). These symmetrical, white skeletal muscles function anaerobically during quick bursts of contraction. A narrow band of aerobic or red skeletal muscle is located superficially between the epaxial and hypaxial musculature beneath the lateral-line canal. This muscle is well vascularized and has a higher fat and myoglobin content and a narrower muscle-fiber diameter than the white muscle (Grizzle and Rogers 1976). It functions primarily during continuous slower swimming. Most other skeletal muscle is attached to skeletal elements and controls fins, opercula, gills and jaw elements (Fig. 23C).

Smooth muscle originates from mesenchyme and is found in the walls of the alimentary tract, swim bladder, gall bladder, urinary bladder, go-

---

Figure 25. Muscular system of striped bass.

A. Skeletal muscle fibers, 3-year-old fish (formalin; H&E). Bar = 8.8 μm.
B. Transverse section of skeletal muscle bundles, 3-year-old fish (formalin; H&E). Bar = 6.6 μm.
C. Sagittal section of the dorsal musculature, 3-month-old fish (formalin; H&E). Bar = 45 μm.
D. Oblique section of the epaxial myomeres, 3-month-old fish (formalin; H&E). Bar = 45 μm.
E. Longitudinal muscle layer of the intestines, 3-year-old fish (Bouin's; H&E). Bar = 29 μm.
F. Cardiac muscle fibers of the ventricle, 3-year-old fish (formalin; H&E). Bar = 9.2 μm.

1 A-bands
2 Central nucleus
3 Dorsal fin depressor
4 Dorsal fin erector
5 Endothelial nuclei
6 Epaxial myomeres
7 I-bands
8 Intercellular space and the endomysium
9 Lepidotrichia
10 Myelinated nerve fibers
11 Myosepta (myocommata)
12 Peripheral nucleus
13 Red blood cell
14 Serosa
15 Skeletal muscle fibers

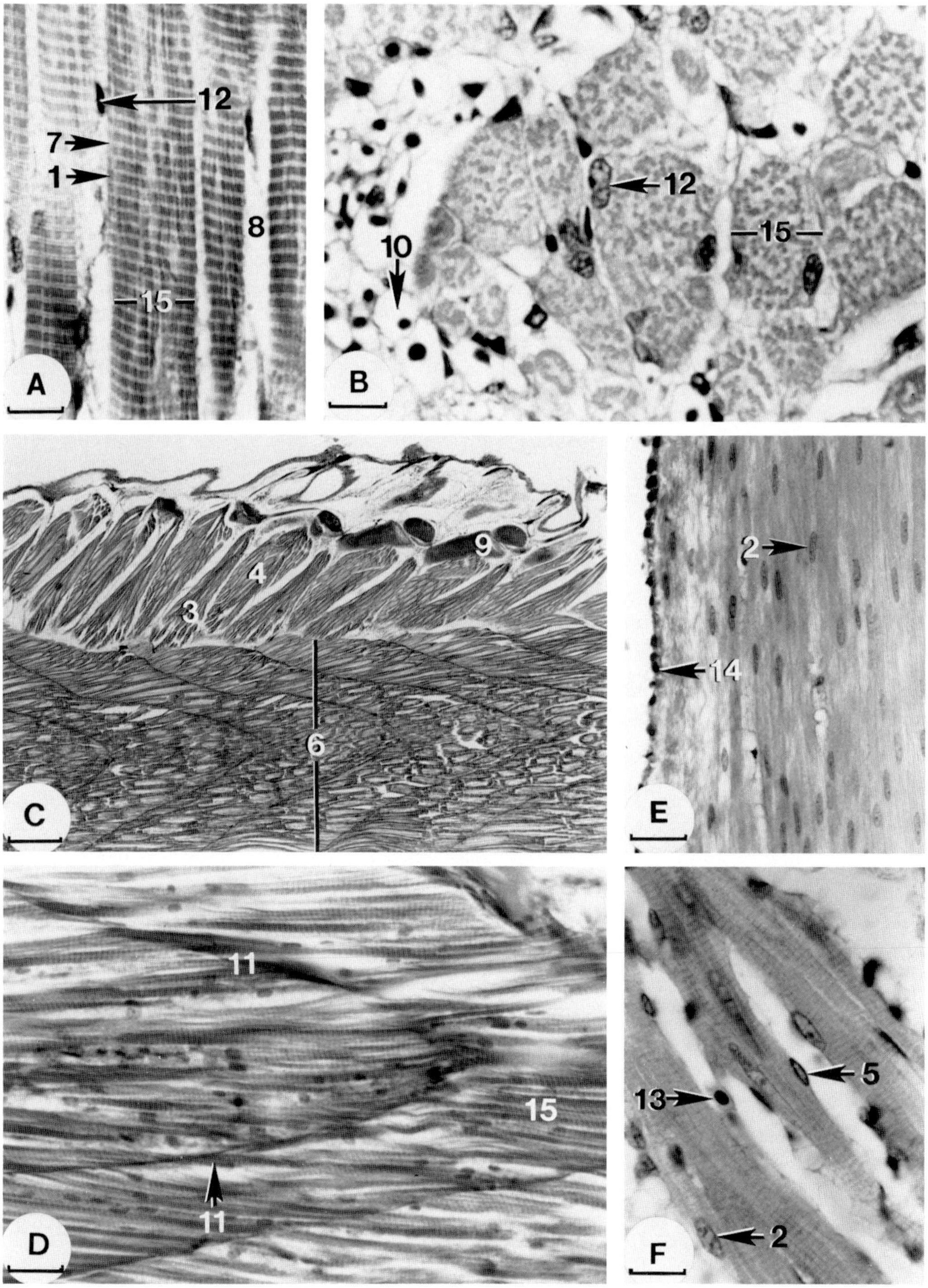

Figure 25

nads, pancreatic ducts, blood vessels, and structures derived from the above in striped bass. It is not subject to voluntary control, but is regulated by the autonomic nervous system (Harder 1975). Smooth muscle bundles are composed of elongated spindle-shaped cells with centrally placed oval nuclei (Fig. 25E). These cells may occur individually within connective tissue, like the tunica albuginea of the gonads, or in organized circular and longitudinal layers, like the wall of the alimentary tract (Fig. 12C) (Grizzle and Rogers 1976). Unlike skeletal muscle fibers, smooth muscle cells do not contain cross-striations, but do have contractile elements arranged irregularly though parallel to the long axis of the cell. Smooth muscle contracts more slowly than skeletal or cardiac muscle but does not tire as quickly.

Striated cardiac muscle was only found in the heart walls of striped bass. It consists of a complex anastomosing network of fibers that are connected by intercalated discs. This muscle originates from splanchnopleure and is more closely related to smooth muscle than to skeletal muscle (Harder 1975). In particular, the fibers that compose the spongy layer of the heart ventricle are enclosed by a single vascular endothelium (Fig. 4B) (see Circulatory System, page 8). Each fiber contains several centrally located oval nuclei that should not be confused with the flattened peripheral nuclei of the ventricular endothelial lining (Fig. 25F). To keep the blood flowing, cardiac muscle must contract continually, and is under less voluntary control than skeletal muscle.

Figure 26. Skeletal system of striped bass.

A. Transverse section of a neural spine, 3-year-old fish (Bouin's; HPS). Bar = 69 μm.
B. Sagittal section of the neurocranium and enclosed semicircular canals, 3-month-old fish (formalin; H&E). Bar = 188 μm.
C. Developing acellular bone from the nasal region (snout), 3-year-old fish (formol sublimate; H&E). Bar = 23 μm.
D. Sagittal section through the caudal peduncle and fin, 3-month-old fish (formalin; HPS). Bar = 218 μm.
E. Enlargement of the vertebrae and notochord from **D** (formalin; HPS). Bar = 85 μm.
F. Peripheral chondroid of the hypural bones, 3-year-old fish (formalin; H&E). Bar = 9 μm.

1 Acellular bone
2 Amphicoelous centra
3 Caudal fin intraradial muscles
4 Caudal fin superficial flexor muscles
5 Epaxial myomeres
6 Flattened osteoblasts
7 Hyaline cartilage
8 Hypaxial myomeres
9 Hypural bones
10 Lumen of the semicircular canals
11 Macula
12 Notochord
13 Nucleus of a chondroid cell
14 Osteoblast
15 Pars hyporals
16 Prezygapophysis (articulating vertebral process)
17 Spinal ganglion
18 Vertebra

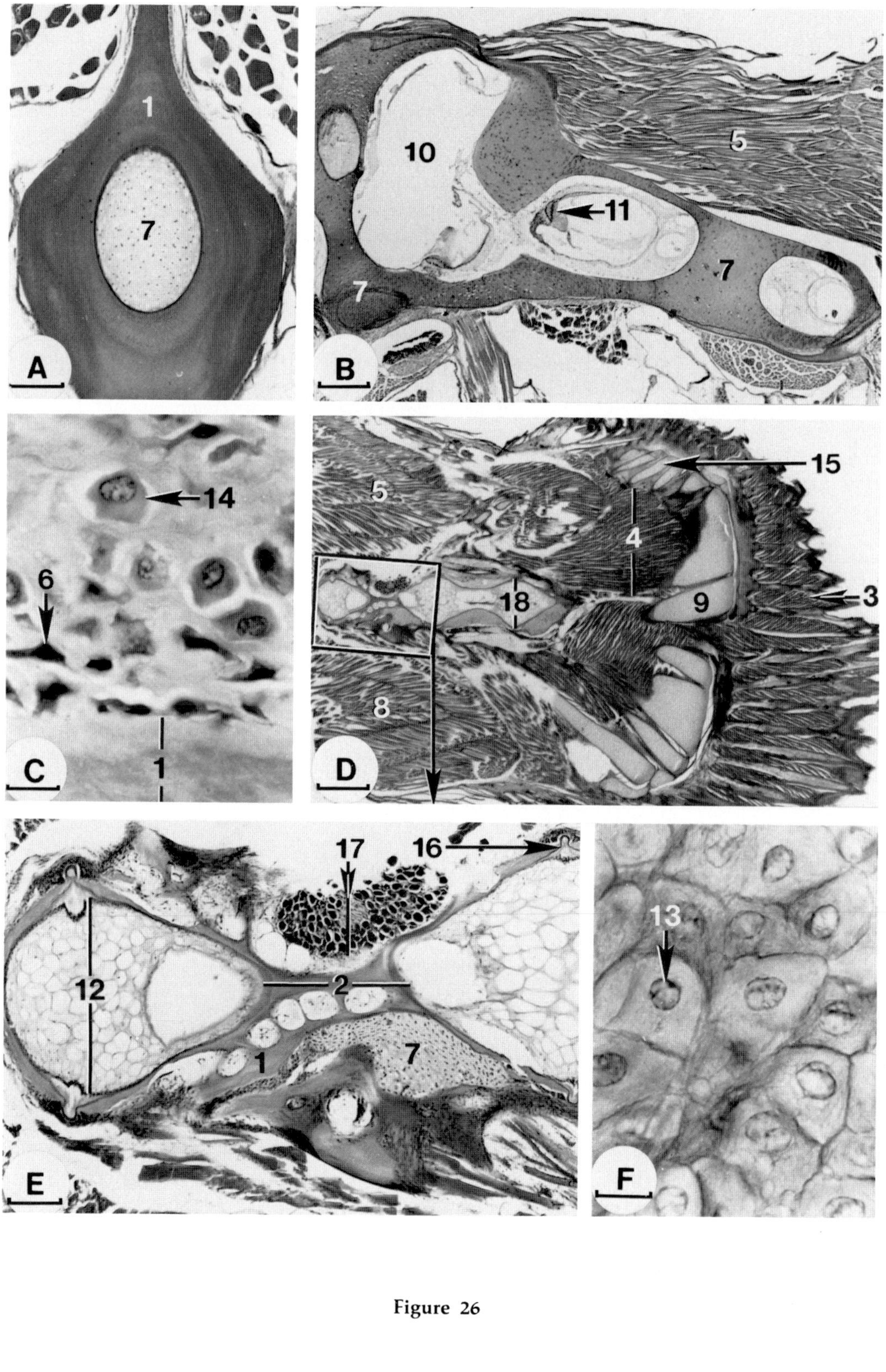

Figure 26

Skeletal System

The osteology of the striped bass was thoroughly examined by Merriman (1940) and Woolcott (1957); Figure 2 shows an X-ray image of skeletal elements. Any further discussion in this study of the skeletal element will be confined to the histology and not to specific osteology.

Fish, like all vertebrates, have axial skeleton bone and cartilage that provide a frame for the body musculature, protect major organs like the brain, and are involved with calcium metabolism, primarily as a source of stored ions (Weiss and Watabe 1978). Body tissues are attached to the skeleton by connective-tissue elements. With the exception of the notochord, intercellular substances make up most of this connective tissue (Harder 1975). In addition to its axial portion (vertebral column and skull), the skeleton has dermal elements (teeth, and other membranous bones of the head) and appendicular elements (spines and lepidotrichia) that were discussed as part of the integumentary system.

Harder (1975) noted that teleosts have more kinds of supporting tissues and tissues intermediate between cartilage and bone than any other group of vertebrates. The formation of teleost bone from cartilaginous elements occurs both by direct ossification, as in dermal or membranous bone, and by indirect perichondral and endochondral ossification of hyaline cartilage, as occurs for chondral bone. Perichondral ossification results in structures (neural and hemal spines) having a core of cartilage surrounded by acellular bone (Figure 26A), whereas endochondral ossification forms the major bones of the axial skeleton (neurocranium, vertebrae, et cetera) which are acellular (Fig. 26B).

In higher bony fishes like the striped bass, all acellular bone is surrounded by a periosteum composed of a fibrous connective tissue layer and an osteogenic layer. The latter contains osteoblasts that secrete the collagenous ground substance of acellular bone (Harder 1975). Osteoblasts are irregularly shaped acidophilic cells and contain large rounded nuclei with diffuse chromatin (Fig. 26C). They are widely spaced within newly formed ground substance, become flattened and degenerate distal to the periosteum, and are absent in the acellular bony matrix. In striped bass, acellular bone constitutes a major portion of amphicoelous vertebral centra, the basic elements of the vertebral column (Fig. 1, 2). These centra resemble biconical hour-glass-shaped cylinders (Fig. 26D,E), the ends of which are concave in teleosts (Laerm 1976). Each centrum contains articulating zygapophyseal processes that increase the area of contact between adjacent vertebrae (Fig. 26E). In addition, spongy bone and hyaline cartilage surround the compact centra to form longitudinal bars along its lateral margins.

A rod-shaped notochord is situated within the vertebral column from the neurocranium to the root of the caudal fin. In bony fish, it is constricted at regular intervals by the biconical centra (Fig. 26E) and is surrounded by a single-celled connective-tissue sheath. According to Harder (1975), the notochord is composed of chondroid, a noncalcareous tissue intermediate between cartilage and

---

Figure 27. Skeletal system of striped bass.

A. Transverse section of a vertebra, the notochord (ventral), and the spinal cord (dorsal), 3-month-old (formalin; HPS). Bar = 57 μm.
B. Notochord and vertebral bone, 3-year-old fish (formalin; HPS). Bar = 60 μm.
C. Mixed bone of the skull, 3-year-old fish (formol sublimate; HPS). Bar = 41 μm.
D. Cartilage of the gill filaments, 3-year-old fish (Helly's; HPS). Bar = 5.3 μm.

1 Acellular bone
2 Adipose tissue
3 Chondrocyte
4 Chondroid-like cells of notochord
5 Connective tissue sheath
6 Dense connective tissue
7 Dorsal horn (gray matter)
8 Extracellular cartilaginous matrix
9 Hyaline cartilage
10 Intracellular cartilaginous matrix
11 Kidney tissue
12 Mauthner axons
13 Myelinated nerve axons (white matter)
14 Periosteum
15 Pseudo-Haversian canals
16 Sheath of the notochord
17 Skeletal muscle bundles
18 Vacuoles
19 Ventral horns (gray matter)

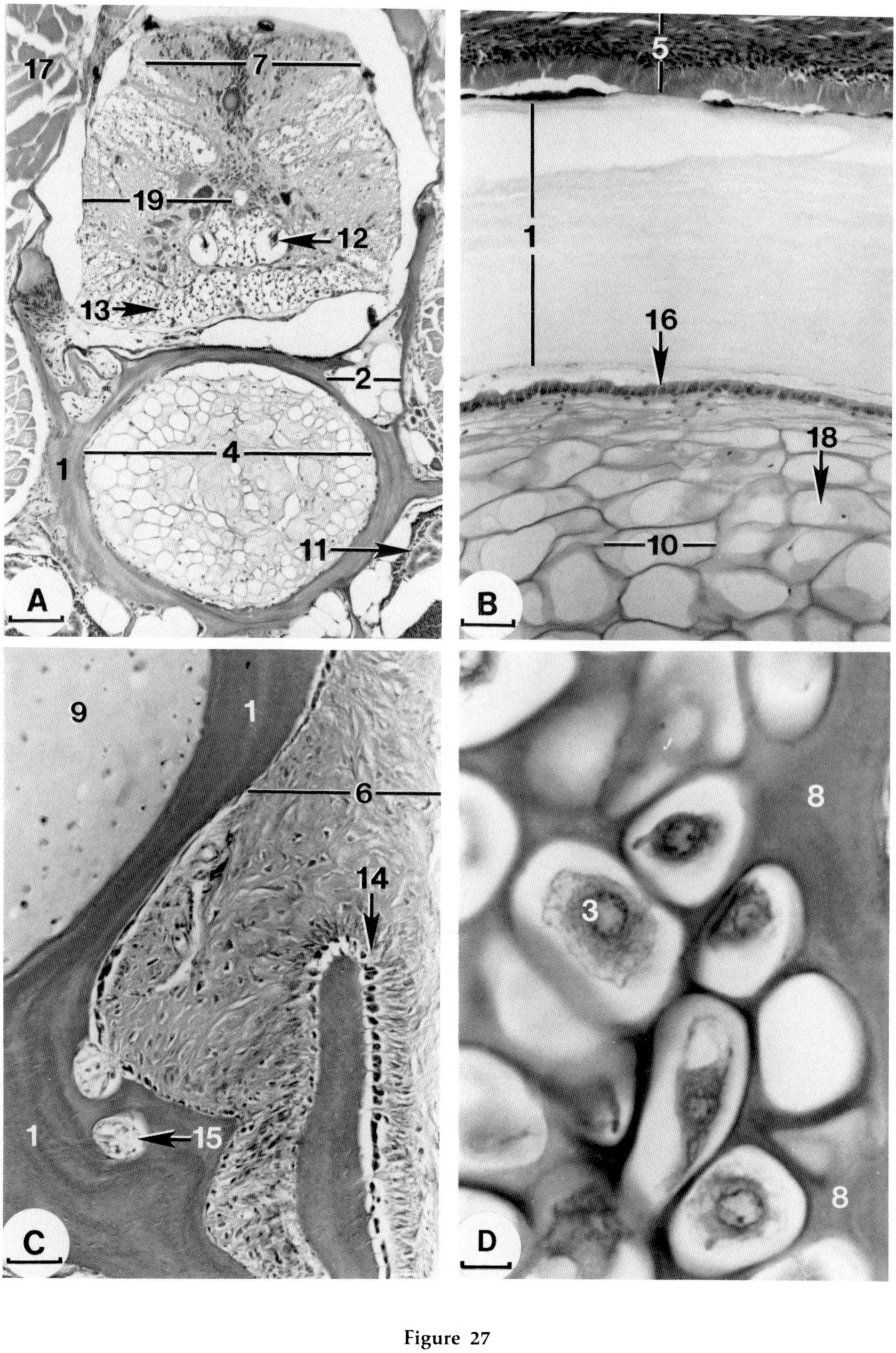

Figure 27

cellular connective tissue, whose turgescent cells contain fluid-filled vacuoles (intracellular matrix) that displace other nuclear and cytoplasmic elements to the cell periphery (Figs. 26F, 27A,B). Grizzle and Rogers (1976) contend that the notochord cells (Fig. 27B) are different from true condroid (Fig. 26F) because they contain an intracellular matrix unlike cartilage or bone. In striped bass, chondroid also surrounds the dermal bone of the tongue and the hypural bones of the caudal fin. The large irregularly shaped acidophilic chondroid cells are separated from one another by scattered intercellular fibers, contain no vacuolated intracellular matrix, and have rounded central nuclei with diffuse chromatin (Fig. 26E).

Bone containing several cartilagenous-skeletal or connective-tissue elements is termed mixed bone (Fig. 27C). It is formed by the fusion of dermal and chondral bony elements and may contain hyaline cartilage, acellular bone, and areolar and dense connective tissue. Mixed bone has a distinct periosteum with spindle-shaped cartilage cells (Fig. 27C) and irregular osteoblasts (Fig. 26C) that separates the acellular bone from surrounding connective tissue and melanocytes (Harder 1975). Spongy bone, a specific type of mixed teleost bone, is laminated and contains spaces that give it a porous or spongy appearance. In addition to being located proximal to the vertebrae, mixed bone and spongy bone occur in association with jaw bones (Fig. 8B), gill arch bones (Fig. 17C), and other cephalic skeletal elements of striped bass. The blood vessels that supply teleost bone occur in strands of connective tissue; these strands originate from the periosteum or surrounding connective tissue layer, but may also occur together with areolar connective tissue in spongy bone, forming simple pseudo-Haversian canals (Fig. 27C) (Grizzle and Rogers 1976).

The skull is the anterior portion of the axial skeleton and contains both neurocranial and branchiocranial elements. The neurocranium shelters and supports the brain and larger sensory organs (olfactory apparatus, eyes, inner ear). In addition, the ventral continuation of the neurocranium (visceral cranium) supports the anterior-most section of the digestive tract. In juvenile striped bass, the axial skeleton including the skull is preformed by hyaline cartilage or true basophilic cartilage (Fig. 26B), the chondrocytes of which are suspended within an abundant watery intercellular substance containing a high content of chondromucoids. In adult striped bass, much of the cartilage becomes mineralized, forming chondral bone, dermal bone, and mixed bone such as that found in the ethmoid region of the neurocranium (Fig. 27C).

Special gill-ray cartilage also is present in gills of striped bass. Unlike the basophilic hyaline cartilage, its intercellular matrix stains acidophilically. This smooth cartilage contains large, often rectangular, basophilic chondrocytes that are separated by less intercellular matrix than those of hyaline cartilage (Fig. 27D). Ossification of the gill-ray cartilage occurs proximal to the mixed bones of the gill arch, according to Grizzle and Rogers (1976).

No pseudocartilage as described by Grizzle and Rogers (1976) for channel catfish was found in the striped bass. However, acrodont teeth, which form from the dermal skeleton of the head, are present (see Digestive System, page 22).

Nervous System

The nervous system of vertebrates primarily functions in the rapid transmission of information. In teleosts, as in other vertebrates, it correlates this information to enable the organism to orient itself in the surrounding environment, to integrate control of the organism's internal environment, and to facilitate learning (Harder 1975).

The basic structure of the teleost nervous system includes neurons, glial cells, ependymal-lining cells, astrocytes, phagocytic Hartega cells (macrophages), vascular elements, epithelial elements such as those comprising the meninx primitiva and tela choroidea, and non-neuronal ectodermal and dural supporting tissues (Ariens Kappers et al. 1965; Harder 1975; Pearson and Pearson 1976). These tissues are organized into central and peripheral components. The central nervous system includes the brain and the spinal cord. The peripheral nervous system (autonomic) consists of mixed nerve-fiber bundles and ganglia (sympathetic and parasympathetic), which are most apparent along the spinal nerves (Fig. 28A). The mixed nerve fibers have both myelinated and unmyelinated portions (Fig. 28B,C); the ganglia are composed of large multinucleated nerve cells and nerve fibers (Figs. 28D, 12F). The sympathetic ganglia are adjacent to the spinal cord (Fig. 26E) whereas the parasympathetic ganglia are located close to or inside effector organs, the Plexus of Auerbach, for example (Fig. 12F) (Campbell and Gannon, 1976).

The central nervous system integrates stimuli from sensory organs, and directs reactions to them. The spinal cord may control locomotion independently of the brain. In the striped bass, as with other teleosts, the spinal cord and the brain share common structural elements: nerve tracts; nuclei; meninx primitiva; and the ependymal cell linings of the ventricles. The spinal cord, however, is structurally less complex than the brain, which commonly is subdivided by embryonic regions: myelencephalon; metencephalon; mescencephalon; diencephalon; and telencephalon.

Myelencephalon

The myelencephalon comprises the rostral region of the brain and contains the medulla oblongata (Fig. 29A) that integrates the reticulomotor system and taste and auditory senses (Lagler et al. 1977). In the striped bass, the central canal is enlarged where it forms the fossa rhomboidea or fourth ventricle in the caudal medulla oblongata (Fig. 29B). This ventricle is also lined by ependymal cells and has a thin dorsal roof or velum posticum. The rostral section of the velum is well vascularized and forms the tela choroidea posterior, which supplies the ventricle with cerebrospinal fluid. Paired vagal lobes are evident in the dorsal medulla oblongata (Fig. 29B); however, neither these nor the more rostral facial lobes are very prominent. This may suggest that the striped bass does not rely as heavily on taste to acquire food as channel catfish (Grizzle and Rogers 1976). According to Harder (1975), several cranial nerves (oculomotor III, trochlear IV, trigeminal V, abducens VI, facial VII, acoustic VIII, glossopharyngeal IX, and vagus X) in addition to the first spinal nerve (hypoglossus XII) originate from the medulla oblongata.

Metencephalon

The metencephalon contain the cerebellum, valvula cerebelli, and their associated nerve tracts. The cerebellum in fish has been thoroughly discussed by Nieuwenhuys (1967) and Pouwells (1976). It integrates information concerned with postural reflexes, maintenance of muscle tone, and stimuli from the eyes and acoustico-lateralis organs (Grizzle and Rogers 1976). In striped bass, the cerebellum is divided into a prominent corpus cerebelli and moderately lobed valvula cerebelli (Fig. 29A). The corpus cerebelli has a neck region extending caudodorsad from the medulla oblongata just rostral to the facial lobes, and a head region extending both rostrally over the optic tectum and caudally over the velum posticum. The cerebellum contains an outer molecularis primarily comprised of dendritic fibers. It is covered by the meninx primitiva and an inner granular layer, made up of neuronal perikarya, which lacks any distinguishable remnant of the fourth ventricle. The granular layer develops into a prominent eminentia granularis (Pouwells 1976) that extends out over the fossa rhomboidea at that point in the neck of the corpus where the molecular layer is quite thin (Fig. 29C). Lying between the molecularis and granularis is a band of Purkinje cells (Fig. 29D), which have long dendritic processes that synapse with the dendrites and axons of other neurons in the molecularis (Harder 1975).

The valvula cerebelli is formed by an invagination of the molecularis and granularis into the third ventricle (ventriculus mesencephali). It contains two dorsolateral lobes and one ventral lobe in which the molecular and granular layers appear reversed in relation to those of the corpus (Figs. 29E, 30A,B,C). Rostrally, the dorsal lobes press upward against the torus longitudinalis. An epithelial layer or tela mesencephalica covers the valvula, forming plica (Fig. 30C) between the dorsal and ventral lobes. The Purkinje cells are well developed in the valvula cerebelli and the entire structure lies beneath the optic tectum and is contained within the third ventricle.

Mesencephalon

The mesencephalon is the largest section of the striped bass brain and primarily receives and integrates visual stimuli from the eyes. It has a prominently layered optic tectum and a less complex tegumentum (Fig. 29A). The optic tectum is the main optic center, being the most important center of nervous integration for piscivorous fish like striped bass that primarily use sight to obtain food.

Externally, the optic tectum appears as two optic lobes that join along the sagittal plane of the brain. At this point the medial part of the stratum periventriculare extends into the third ventricle as a paired torus longitudinalis (Figs. 29E, 30D,E), which is thicker at the rostral end where it joins the posterior commissura. This structure receives myelinated afferent fibers from varying portions of the brain and sends unmyelinated efferent fibers to the molecularis of the optic tectum (Harder 1976). The torus longitudinalis functions to help adjust the position of the body in space. Both structures are covered externally by a well-vascularized meninx primitiva and internally by the tela mesencephalica, which borders on the third ventricle.

The layers of the optic tectum have been discussed by Arien Kappers et al. (1965) and Harder (1975). The striped bass has six histologically distinguishable layers (Fig. 31A,B): stratum marginale; stratum opticum; stratum fibrosum et griseum superficiale; stratum album centrale; stratum griseum centrale; stratum periventriculare. These layers have different neuron concentration and afferent fiber connections. The tela mesencephalica, which contains ciliated ependymal cells (Fig. 31C), is not regarded as a distinct layer.

At the base of the optic lobes is the torus semicircularis (Fig. 30A) composed of lateral and central nuclei that together form the dorsal border of the tegumentum (Fig. 30B,D). These nuclei also are covered by the tele mesencephalica. The fourth ventricle is connected to the third via the mesencephalic aqueduct (Sylvian aqueduct), which penetrates through the metencephalon to the tegumentum ventrad to the valvular cerebelli (Figs. 29E, 30C).

Diencephalon

The diencephalon receives primary olfactory information from the telencephalon and processes it together with gustatory and optic information from other sections of the brain. It maintains an intimate neural connection with all other portions of the central nervous system and contains appendages whose functions are completely different from those of the rest of the brain; these appendages include the pituitary gland, the pineal organ, the pariental organ or saccus dorsalis, and

---

Figure 28. Nervous system of striped bass.

A. Transverse section of a vertebral centrum and spinal ganglion, 3-year-old fish (formalin; H&E). Bar = 255 μm.
B. Sagittal section of a mixed cranial nerve, 3-year-old fish (formol sublimate; H&E). Bar = 44 μm.
C. Transverse section of a mixed cranial nerve, 3-year-old fish (formalin; H&E). Bar = 63 μm.
D. Autonomic ganglion proximal to pancreatic tissue, 3-year-old fish (Helly's; PTAH). Bar = 42 μm.
E. Sagittal section of the spinal cord dorsal to the trunk kidney in a 3-month-old fish (formalin; H&E). Bar = 212 μm.

1 Adipose tissue
2 Blood vessel
3 Dorsal aorta
4 Intestine
5 Multinucleated ganglion cells
6 Myelinated nerve fibers
7 Nerve fibers (mixed)
8 Nonmyelinated nerve fibers
9 Notochord
10 Perineurium
11 Posterior cardinal vein
12 Skeletal muscle bundles
13 Spinal cord
14 Stomach
15 Trunk kidney
16 Vertebral bone

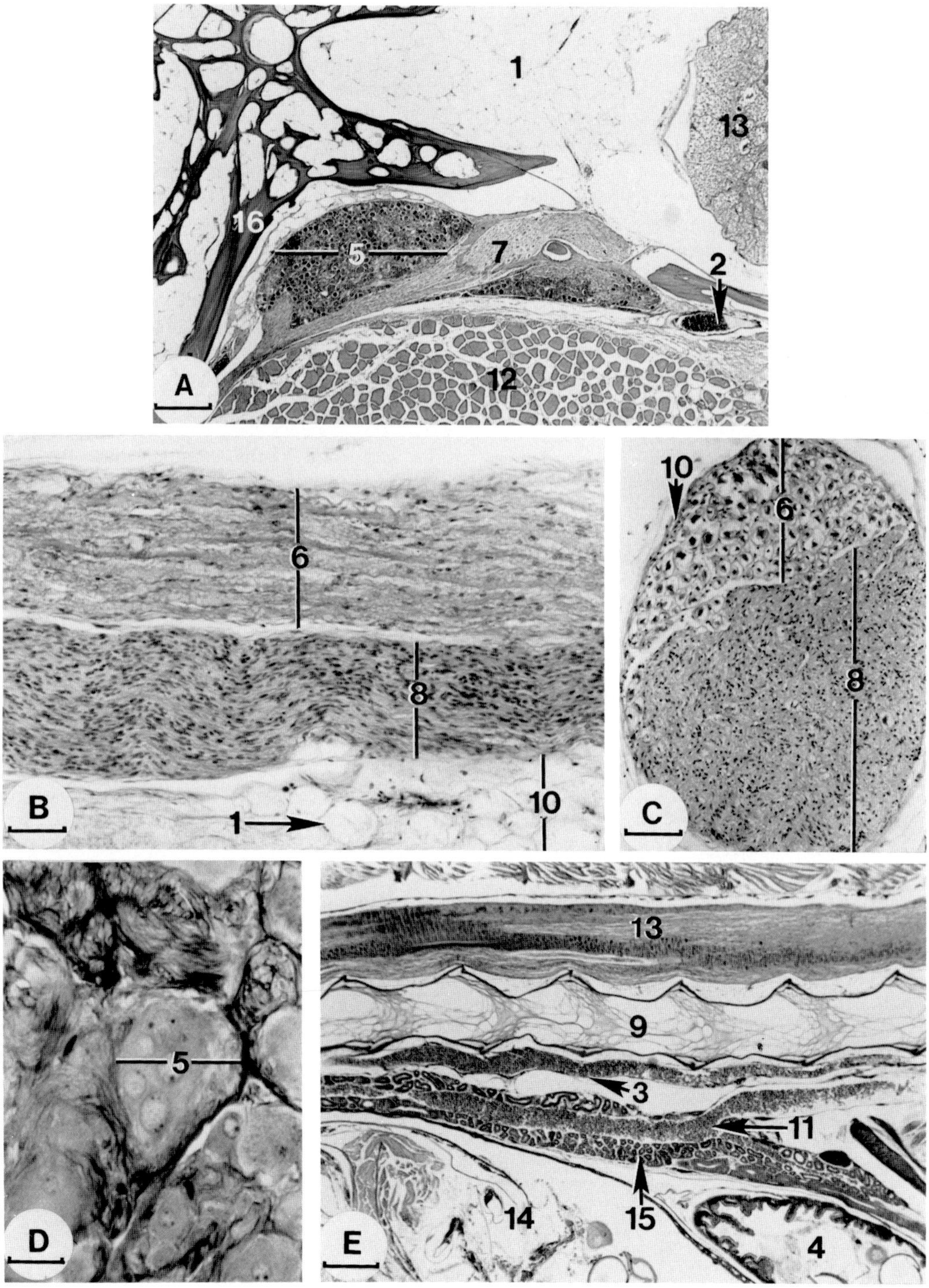

Figure 28

the saccus vasculosus. The diencephalon has three regions: epithalamus; thalamus; hypothalamus.

Epithalamus

The epithalamus contains the pineal organ, saccus dorsalis, parts of the posterior commissura, habenular ganglia, associated nuclei, and fiber tracts (Figs. 31D,E, 32A,B). The flattened pineal organ is dorsal to the telencephalon and lies against the dorsal cranium. Its comparative morphology in teleosts has been well described (Hafeez 1971; McNulty 1976; McNulty and Nafpaktitis 1977). In striped bass, this organ is suspended rostral to the rest of the diencephalon by a hollow stalk that originates proximal to the habenular ganglia. Both the stalk and the pineal organ are surrounded by meninges and a highly vascularized connective-tissue capsule. This vascular system also supplies the endomeninx of the saccus dorsalis (Fig. 32B). Hafeez (1971) included the striped bass in a histological study of the pineal organ in teleosts. He noted some attenuation of the lumen at the junction of the pineal vesicle and stalk where the epithelial folds are most extensive. Neurones or neuron-like cells generally are located in the basal part of the luminal epithelium, according to Hafeez (1971). These neurones are large cells with abundant cytoplasm and a large nucleus containing a prominent nucleolus. In addition to epithelial and neural elements, the pineal contains distinct primary sensory cells and supporting cells in the parenchyma. The sensory cells occur close to the lumen; each contains a large basal nucleus and an apical process (Hafeez 1971). The supporting cells occur throughout the epithelium of the pineal organ, but are most abundant in its basal portion. They have little cytoplasm and an irregular nucleus. It is generally accepted that the sensory cells are photosensitive, thus suggesting photoreception as the primary function of the pineal organ.

The saccus dorsalis is the dorsorostral evagination of the diencephalon roof and is composed of a meninx primitiva and ciliated cuboidal epithelium. The lumen of the saccus dorsalis is continuous with the pineal stalk, the third ventricle, and the tela choroidea of the common ventricle, which covers part of the telencephalon (Fig. 32C). In striped bass, as in rainbow trout, the folded wall of the saccus dorsalis is connected to the habenular ganglia and separates the cerebrospinal fluid from the meningeal matrix fluid (Jansen$_1$ et al. 1976). Jansen$_2$ et al. (1976) presented evidence for this organ's involvement in fluid secretion, extrusion of low-molecular-weight organic substances into the ventricular system, uptake of high-molecular-

Figure 29. Nervous system of striped bass.

A. Sagittal section of the brain, 3-month-old fish (formalin; H&E). Bar = 141 μm.
B. Transverse section of the caudal myelencephalon (medulla oblongata), 3-month-old fish (formalin; H&E). Bar = 121 μm.
C. Transverse section of the metencephalon (cerebellum and medulla oblongata), 3-month-old fish (Bouin's; H&E). Bar = 282 μm.
D. Sagittal section of the cerebellum, 3-year-old fish (formol sublimate; H&E). Bar = 60 μm.
E. Transverse section of the rostral metencephalon, 3-year-old fish (Bouin-Allen's; H&E). Bar = 889 μm.

1 Central canal
2 Cerebellum (corpus cerebelli)
3 Cranium
4 Eminentia granularis (granular eminence)
5 Foramen magnum
6 Fourth ventricle
7 Granular cell layer
8 Habenular ganglion
9 Inferior lobe of the hypothalamus
10 Infundibular recess
11 Intertectal commissure
12 Mauthner's axons
13 Medial lobe of the hypothalamus
14 Medial longitudinal fasiculus
15 Medulla oblongata
16 Mesencephalic aqueduct (Sylvian aqueduct)
17 Molecular cell layer
18 Olfactory lobe (telencephalon)
19 Optic chiasma
20 Optic nerve
21 Optic tectum
22 Periventricular hypothalamic region
23 Pituitary (hypophysis)
24 Preoptic nucleus
25 Preoptic recess
26 Principal granular layer
27 Principal molecular layer
28 Purkinje cells
29 Rostral medulla oblongata
30 Saccus vasculosus
31 Semicircular (stato-acoustic) canals
32 Tegmentum
33 Third ventricle
34 Torus longitudinalis
35 Vagal lobe
36 Valvula cerebelli
37 Ventral molecular layer

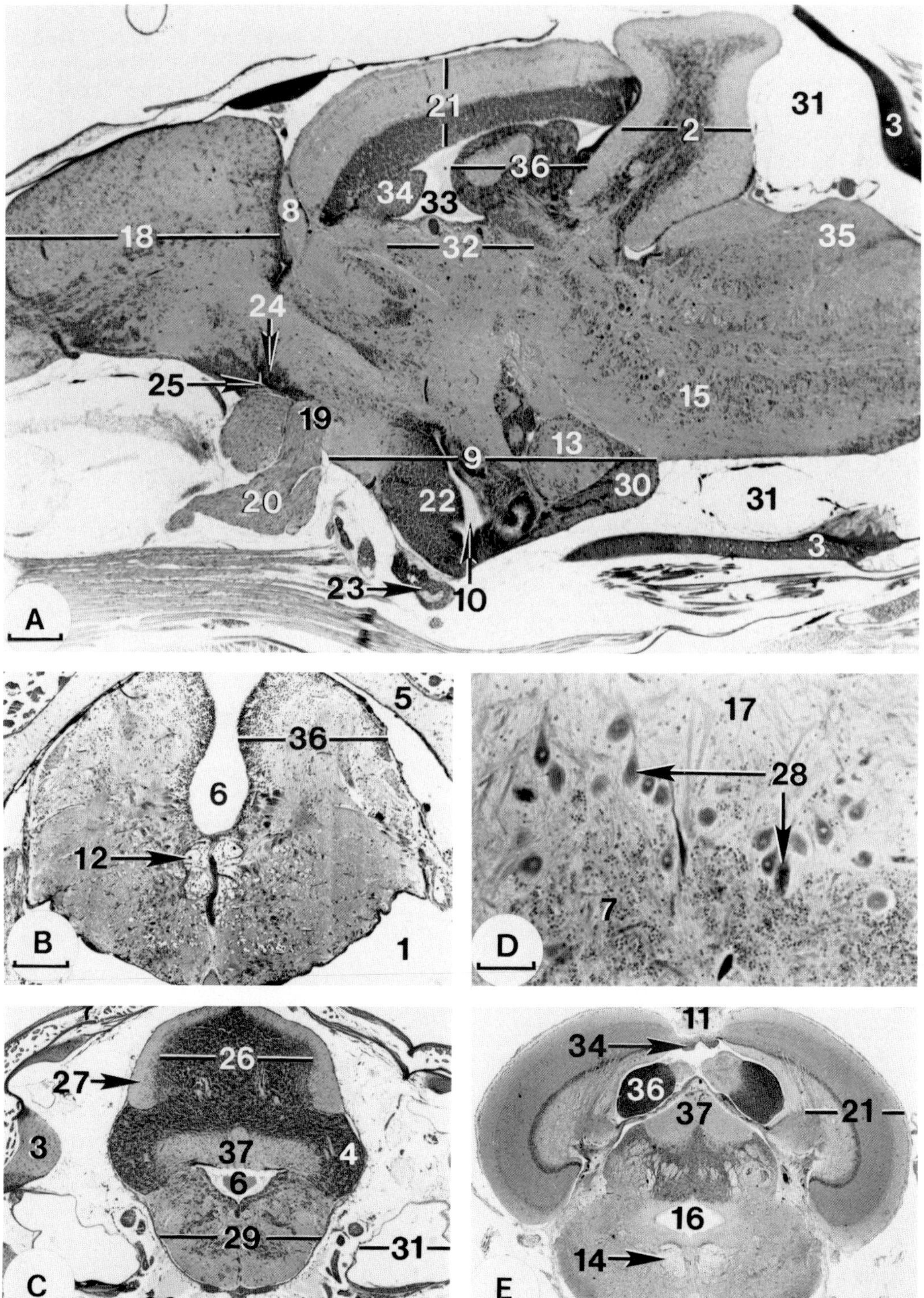
A
21
2
31
3
36
34
33
8
18
32
35
24
25
19
15
13
9
30
20
22
31
3
23
10
B
5
36
6
12
1
D
17
28
7
C
26
27
3
37
4
6
29
31
30
E
11
34
36
37
21
16
14

Figure 29

weight substances, and uptake of low-molecular-weight organic substances from the cerebrospinal fluid.

In striped bass, the bilateral habenular nucleus is caudoventral to the pineal organ (Fig. 31D,E), being contiguous with the rostral mesencephalon and the rostral thalamus (Schnitzlein 1962). Fibers from the saccus dorsalis and the telencephalon lead into this nucleus and provide the dominant nervous interconnection between the olfactory center of the forebrain and various somatomotoric nuclei, according to Harder (1975). The posterior commissura (Fig. 30E) lies caudal to the habenular ganglia and forms the border between the epithalamus and the mesencephalon.

Thalamus

The teleost thalamus forms the lateral borders of the diencephalon and is divided into a dorsal and a ventral region by the subhabenular sulcus (sulcus medius). The dorsal thalamus (Schnitzlein 1962) or posthabenular region contains many nuclei, such as the lateral genicular nuclei and the nucleus rotondus (Fig. 31D,E). Together with other diencephalon centers, the thalamus correlates exteroceptive and proprioceptive sensations and establishes phototactic and gravitactic impulses (Harder 1975).

Hypothalamus

The hypothalamus is the dominant portion of the diencephalon. Its nuclei and comparative structure in fish are discussed by Crosby and Showers (1969). In striped bass, it extends from the optic chiasma (Figs. 29A, 31D) caudad along the ventral diencephalon, forming the infundibular region (medial lobe) and two prominent lateral or inferior lobes (Figs. 30A, 32D). An extensive network of ventricular processes extends throughout the hypothalamus; infundibular recess; lateral recesses; rostral infundibular recess; preoptic recess (Figs. 29, 30). In addition, a large number of sensory and neurosecretory nuclei (preoptic nucleus, mammilary complex, lateral tuberal nucleus, lateral nuclei of the infundibular recess, glomerular nucleus, and magnocellular preoptic nucleus) (Figs. 30, 31D,E), as well as specialized appendages (saccus vasculosus and pituitary), are innervated to the hypothalamus (Fig. 30B). The hypothalamus is a correlation center for olfactory, gustatory, and other sensory impulses in teleost fish. From this region of the diencephalon, tracts pass to the efferent centers of the medulla oblongata (Harder 1975). The hypothalamus also integrates neurosecretory information originating from the pituitary and neurohypophysis (see Endocrine System, page 88).

Figure 30. Brain of striped bass.

- **A.** Transverse section of the caudal mesencephalon and caudal hypothalamus, 3-month-old fish (Bouin's; H&E). Bar = 279 μm.
- **B.** Transverse section of the mid-mesencephalon and hypothalamus, 3-month-old fish (Bouin's; H&E). Bar = 353 μm.
- **C.** Transverse section of the valvula cerebelli (mesencephalon), 3-year-old fish (formal sublimate; H&E). Bar = 267 μm.
- **D.** Transverse section of the mid-rostral mesencephalon and the rostral hypothalamus, 3-month-old fish (Bouin's; H&E). Bar = 276 μm.
- **E.** Transverse section of the rostral mesencephalon and the thalamus–hypothalamus region of the diencephalon, 3-month-old fish (formalin; HPS). Bar = 289 μm.

1 Central nucleus, torus semicircularis
2 Cranium
3 Glomerular nucleus (nucleus glomerulosus)
4 Granular cell layer
5 Inferior lobe of hypothalamus
6 Infundibular recess
7 Lateral lobe of the valvula cerebelli
8 Lateral nuclei of the infundibular recess
9 Lateral nucleus of the torus semicircularis
10 Lateral recess
11 Lateral tuberal nuclei
12 Magnocellular preoptic nucleus
13 Mamillary complex
14 Mesencephalic aqueduct (Sylvian aqueduct)
15 Molecular cell layer
16 Oculomotor nerve
17 Optic tectum
18 Optic tract
19 Pituitary gland
20 Posterior commissura
21 Rostral hypothalamus (infundibulum)
22 Rostral infundibular recess
23 Third ventricle
24 Torus longitudinalis
25 Torus semicircularis
26 Valvula cerebelli
27 Valvular plica
28 Ventral hypothalamus
29 Ventral lobe of the valvula cerebelli

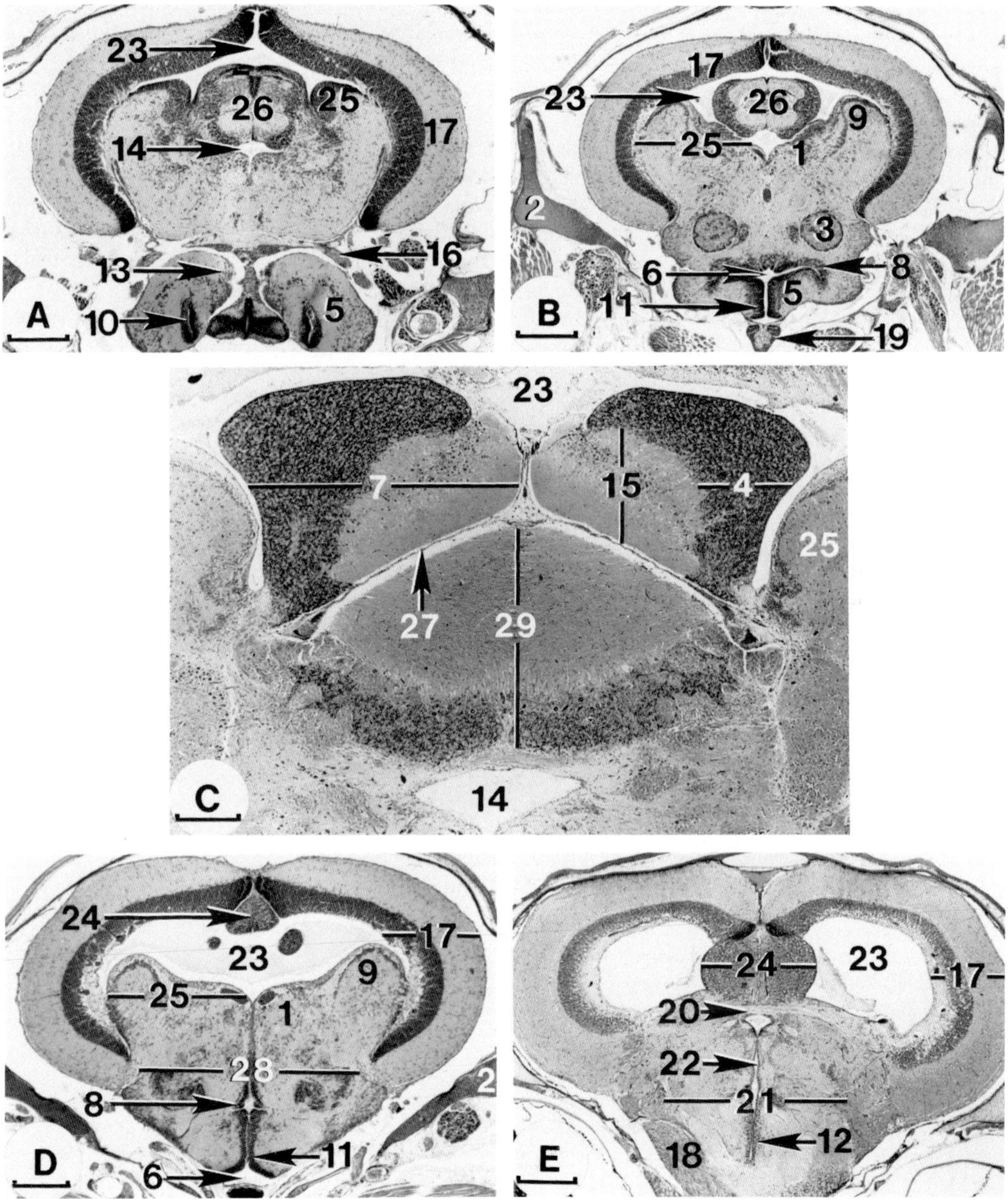
23
26
25
17
14
16
13
A
10
5
17
23
26
9
25
1
2
3
6
8
B
11
5
19
23
7
15
4
25
27
29
C
14
24
17
23
9
25
1
28
2
8
D
11
6
24
23
17
20
22
21
12
18
E

Figure 30

The striped bass saccus vasculosus lies in the caudal hypothalamus between the inferior lobes and posterior to the pituitary (Fig. 32D). This vesicular organ is formed by an evagination of the wall of the infundibulum (Harder 1975). It contains an external meninx primitiva, a highly vascularized endomeninx, and an internal layer of specialized epithelium (Fig. 32E). The meninx primitiva has a well-developed connective-tissue element in which it is common to find macrophages laden with lipofucsin. The endomeninx, in addition to its vascular elements, contains nonmyelinated nerve fibers that, presumably, innervate the specialized epithelium of the internal wall. This wall is extensively folded and borders a lumen that is continuous with the infundibular recess. The epithelium primarily is composed of coronet cells with basally located nuclei and supporting glial cells with apical nuclei (Fig. 32E). The saccus vasculosus may function in the perception of intracerebral liquid pressure, thus aiding the fish to determine depth or, as suggested by Khanna and Singh (1967), it may secrete acid mucopolysaccharides.

The optic chiasma is located between the telencephalon and the rostral diencephalon where the optic nerves cross (Figs. 30E, 29D,E). The optic nerve, therefore, emerges from the diencephalon; however, it is connected to the retina and the optic tectum and only passes through the diencephalon.

Telencephalon

The telencephalon, or cerebrum, of fish is much less significant than that of higher vertebrates, where it is the dominant portion of the brain (Harder 1975). In the striped bass, it consists of paired olfactory lobes and sessile or proximal olfactory bulbs (Figs. 29A, 32A, 33A). The bulbs are connected via afferent nerves to the olfactory organs in the snout. Most of these afferent nerves enter the olfactory lobes by way of fiber tracts that terminate in the epistriatum or ventral area (Fig. 33A). Efferent fibers run from there to the thalamus (Harder 1975).

The bilateral olfactory lobes have five primary areas (Fig. 32A): dorsal; dorsal–lateral; medial; olfactory striatum or somatica; ventral (Meader 1939; Nieuwenhuys 1962, 1963; Schnitzlein 1977). The lobes are connected in the ventral area. The recess that sagitally separates the two lobes is termed the medial ventricle and is the ventral continuation of the common ventricle, which is a union of the first and second ventricles. A portion of the common ventricle forms the roof of the olfactory lobes, consisting of a thin meninx primitiva and a tela choroidea (Fig. 32C). Dorsal to the

---

Figure 31. Brain of striped bass.

A. Sagittal section of the mesencephalon through the optic tectum, 3-year-old fish (formol sublimate; H&E). Bar = 86 μm.
B. Enlargement from the top of **A**. Bar = 46 μm.
C. Enlargement from lower left corner of **A**. Bar = 46 μm.
D. Transverse section through epithalamus (diencephalon), 3-month-old fish (Helly's; H&E). Bar = 133 μm.
E. Transverse section of the thalamic diencephalon, 3-month-old fish (Bouin's; H&E). Bar = 143 μm.
F. Transverse section of the caudal epithalamus and rostral thalamus of the diencephalon, 3-month-old fish (Bouin's; H&E). Bar = 131 μm.

1 Blood vessel
2 Ciliated ependymal cells
3 Cranium
4 Ependymal lining of the third ventricle
5 Granular layer of the valvular cerebelli
6 Habenular ganglion
7 Lateral genicular nucleus
8 Magnocellular preoptic nucleus
9 Meninx primtiva (meninges)
10 Olfactory lobes (telencephalon)
11 Optic chiasma
12 Optic lobe of the mesencephalon
13 Optic tract
14 Pineal organ (epiphysis)
15 Pineal stalk
16 Preoptic nucleus
17 Preoptic recess
18 Saccus dorsalis
19 Stratum album centrale
20 Stratum fibrosum et griseum superficiale
21 Stratum grisum centrale
22 Stratum marginale
23 Stratum opticum
24 Stratum periventriculare
25 Subhabenular sulcus
26 Thalamus
27 Third ventricle
28 Valvula cerebelli

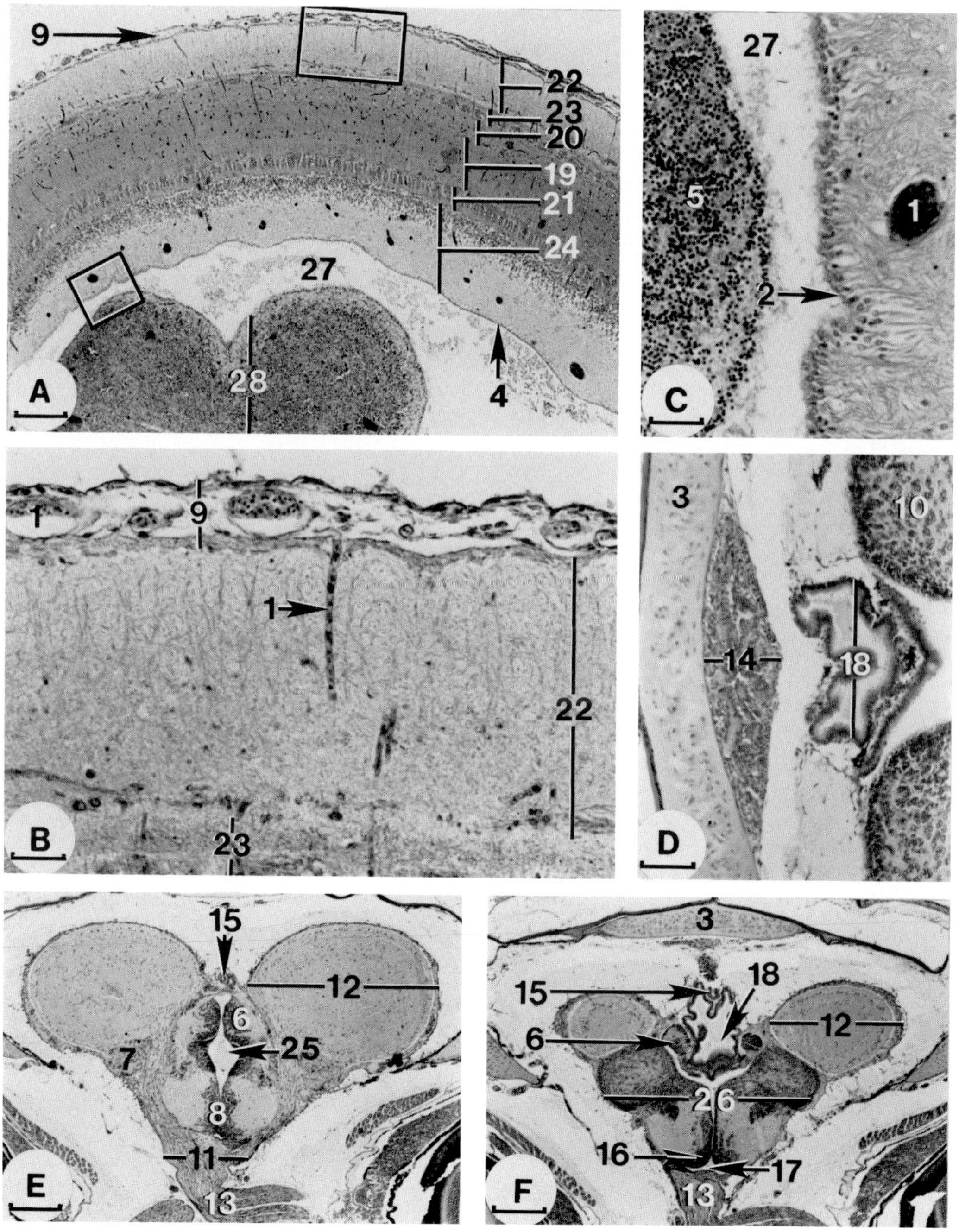

A
9
22
23
20
19
21
24
27
28
4
B
1
9
1
22
23
C
27
5
1
2
D
3
10
14
18
E
15
12
6
25
7
8
11
13
F
3
18
15
6
12
26
16
17
13

Figure 31

optic chiasm, the preoptic recess also penetrates the caudal telencephalon and emerges from the diencephalon, where it is a continuation of the third ventricle. This recess is bordered by the magnocellular preoptic nucleus caudally and the preoptic nucleus rostrally (Fig. 29A).

The telencephalon primarily integrates olfactory stimuli. Grizzle and Rogers (1976), however, indicated that it also may be involved with reproduction, color vision, and learning, and Anderson and Mitchum (1974) add that it may play an important role as an organizer and integrator of innate fish behavior.

Spinal Cord

The spinal cord orginates in the myelencephalon emerging from the cranial cavity through the foramen magnum. It extends the length of the vertebral column to beyond the urophysis (Figs. 1, 28E). The spinal cord is formed by a fusion of its dorsal and ventral roots into a mixed nerve. Such nerves have both myelinated (white matter) and unmyelinated (grey matter) elements. The grey matter of the spinal cord is divided into a dorsal horn and two ventral horns, which are connected and surround a central canal lined by ependymal cells (Fig. 27A). This canal is the caudal continuation of the fourth ventricle of the brain, and also contains cerebral spinal fluid.

The white matter lies between these horns and is best exemplified by the two presumptive Mauthner's fibers found ventral to the central canal. According to Zottoli (1978), in teleost fish these axons (Fig. 29B) probably originate from presumptive Mauthner cells located in the medulla oblongata and follow the longitudinal fasiculus (Fig. 29E) to the spinal cord. At best, we can now state that the Mauthner axons of fish excite ipsilateral motor neurons, and bilaterally activate neurons to the opercula, eyes, and pectoral fin muscles.

The neural canal, formed by the neural arches of the vertebrae, supports and protects the spinal cord, and contains areolar connective tissue that envelopes the leptomeninx of the spinal cord (Plate 3AC). Spinal nerves originate from the cord at predictable intervals to innervate the body segments. Ganglia are situated along the dorsal roots of these mixed spinal nerves (Fig. 28A).

Figure 32. Brain of striped bass

A. Transverse section of the telencephalon midway between the anterior commissure and the habenular ganglia, 3-month-old fish (Bouin's; H&E). Bar = 118 μm.
B. Transverse section of the transitional region between the olfactory bulb and the telencephalon proper, 3-month-old fish (Bouin's; H&E). Bar = 107 μm.
C. Sagittal section of the brain through the epithalamus, 3-year-old fish (Bouin's; H&E). Bar = 44 μm.
D. Surface of the telencephalon, 3-year-old fish (formol sublimate; H&E). Bar = 18 μm.
E. Transverse section of the ventral hypothalamus (diencephalon), 3-year-old fish (Bouin's; H&E). Bar = 207 μm.
F. The saccus vasculosus, 3-year-old fish (formol sublimate; H&E). Bar = 25 μm.

1 Capillary
2 Common ventricle, telencephalon
3 Coronet cells with basal nuclei
4 Cranium
5 Cuboidal epithelium of tela choroidia
6 Dorsal area, olfactory lobe
7 Dorsal-lateral area, olfactory lobe
8 Endomeninx (endomeningeal space)
9 Habenular ganglion region
10 Hypothalamic sulcus
11 Inferior hypothalamic lobe
12 Lateral recess of the third ventricle
13 Lumen of the sulcus vasculosus
14 Medial area of olfactory lobe
15 Medial ventricle (ventricular impar)
16 Neurons
17 Olfactory lobe
18 Olfactory striae (area olfactosomatica)
19 Pineal organ
20 Preoptic nucleus
21 Preoptic recess
22 Red blood cells
23 Saccus dorsalis
24 Saccus vasculosus
25 Supporting glia cells with apical nuclei
26 Tela choroidia
27 Ventral area, olfactory lobe

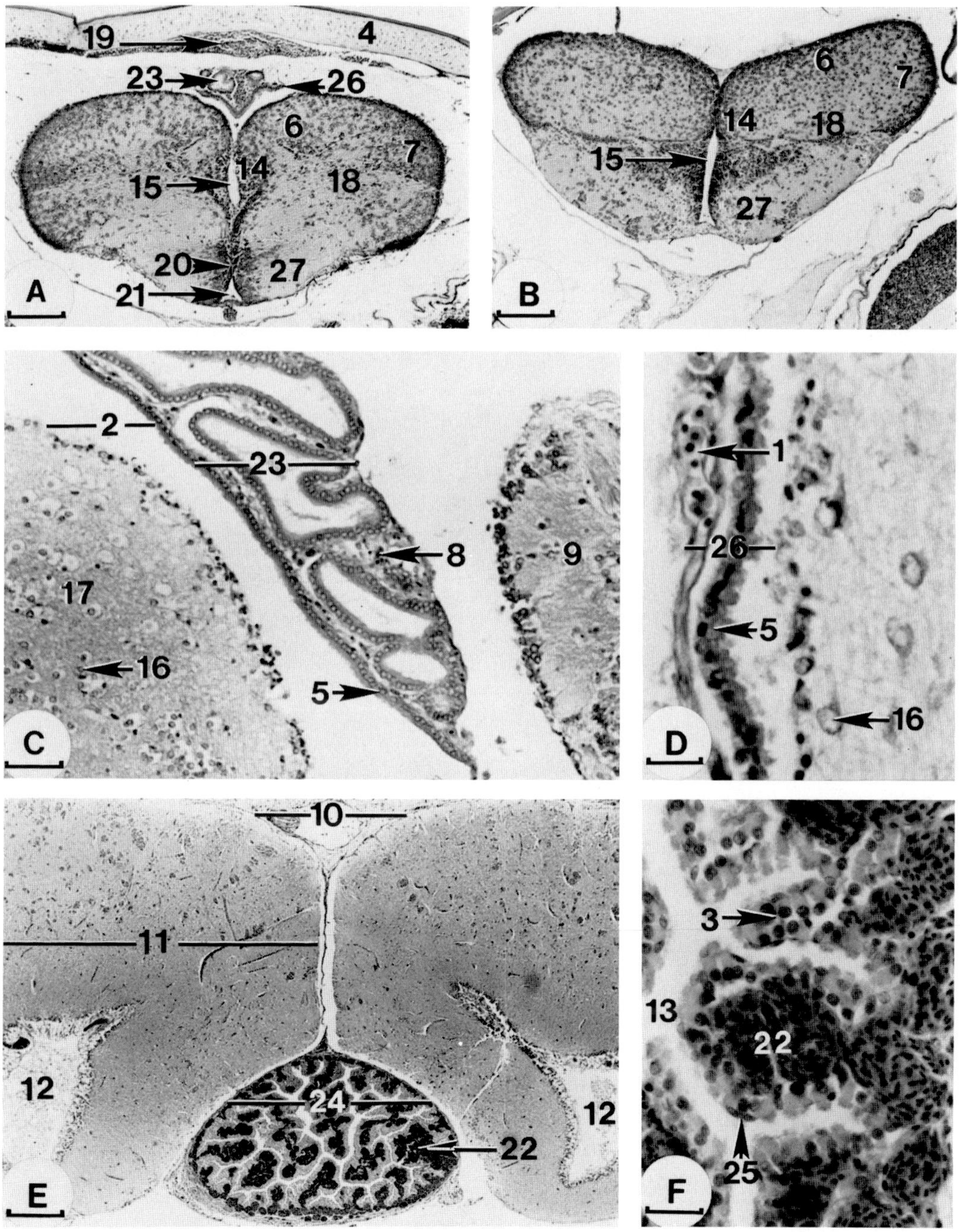
A
19
4
23
26
6
7
15
14
18
20
27
21
B
6
7
14
18
15
27
C
2
23
8
9
17
16
5
D
1
26
5
16
E
10
11
12
24
22
12
F
3
13
22
25

Figure 32

Figure 33. Sensory organs of striped bass.

A. Taste bud of the oral mucosa, 3-year-old fish (formol sublimate; H&E). Bar = 5.6 μm.
B. Oral papillae, 3-year-old fish (Serra's; HPS). Bar = 3.7 μm.
C. Transverse section of a cranial lateral-line canal, 3-month-old fish (formalin; H&E). Bar = 46 μm.
D. Lateral epidermis and musculature of the head, 3-month-old fish (Bouin's; H&E). Bar = 50 μm.
E. Epidermis of the nasal flap, 3-month-old fish (formalin; H&E). Bar = 44 μm.

1 Connective tissue of the sheath
2 Dermal bone
3 Dermis
4 Epidermis
5 Fusiform layer
6 Goblet cells (Type A)
7 Lamina propria
8 Lumen of the buccal cavity
9 Lumen of the lateral-line canal
10 Marginal cells
11 Melanocyte (chromatophore)
12 Nerve plexus
13 Papillary layer of the dermis
14 Sensory cells
15 Skeletal muscle bundles
16 Stratified squamous epithelium
17 Stratum germinativum
18 Superficial neuromast, bell-shaped
19 Superficial neuromast, onion-shaped
20 Sustentacular cells (supporting cells)
21 Taste bud
22 Wandering leukocytes

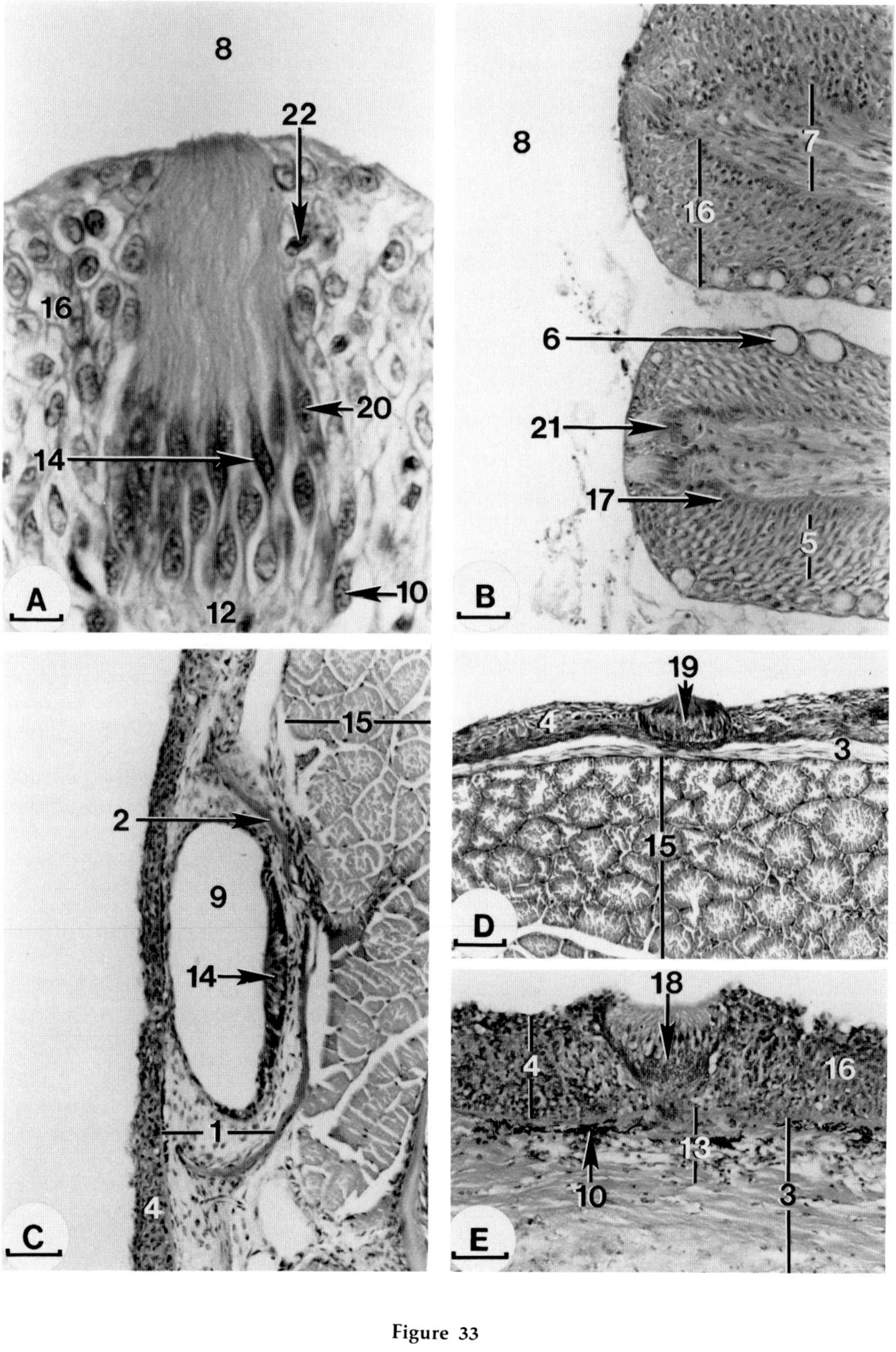
8
22
16
20
14
10
A
12
8
7
16
6
21
17
5
B
19
4
3
15
2
9
14
1
4
C
D
18
4
16
10
13
3
E

Figure 33

Sensory Structures and Organs of Special Sense

Taste Buds

Striped bass have taste buds primarily in the mucosa of the buccal cavity, like those described by Walker et al. (1981) for the fathead minnow (Fig. 33A,B), within the epidermis of the head, and along the mucosa of the gill arches. These simple sensory buds are chemoreceptive and aid in the acquisition of food. Zotterman (1967), in a discussion of the neural mechanism of taste, noted that the taste buds of fish respond strongly to sapid substances, especially phospholipids.

Four epithelial cell types—sensory, basal, sustentacular, and marginal—make up the basic structure of the teleost taste buds (Harder 1975; Walker et al. 1981). Together with the nerve plexus, they form a bulb-shaped neuroepithelial structure that extends from the surface to the basement membrane of the epidermis (Fig. 33A). The cylindrical sensory cells are tightly packed and contain elongated to oval nuclei in their basal thirds. Controversy exists over the number of forms of sensory cells of fish taste buds (Storch and Welsch 1970). Both light- and dark-staining cells have been identified; the former have smooth endoplasmic reticulum and a compact microtubule system, whereas the latter contain a denser cytoplasm with many filaments, dense secretory granules, and a few microtubules, according to Harder (1975). This distinction could not be made by light microscopy for the striped bass. Myelinated taste-bud nerves and a capillary loop extend from the dermis of the skin to the base of the sensory cells, forming the cutis-papilla. Indistinct basal cells also are located in this region, whereas the sustentacular and marginal cells occur more laterally to support the sensory cells and separate them from the rest of the epithelium (Harder 1975) (Fig. 33A). Taste buds are innervated by the facial nerve (VII), glossopharyngeal nerve (IX), and vagus nerve (X).

Lateral-Line Organ

The functional receptors of the lateral-line system are the sensory hillocks or neuromasts that occur either in organized canal systems or superficially in the epidermis (Harder 1975). In either case, these receptors differ markedly from those of the taste buds, by having sustentacular elements located between sensory cells. In striped bass, lateral-line canals occur on the caudal fin, body, trunk, and cranium. The bilateral trunk canals extend from the tail to the opercular region, and are located within the horizontal myoseptal dermis, between the hypaxial and epaxial musculature and beneath specialized scales (Walker 1967; Harder 1975); these scales have pores that connect the canal neuromasts with the external environment. The highly developed cranial canal system is continuous with the rostral end of the trunk canal system. As noted by Reno (1966) for the mimic shiner, the lateral-line canals on the head of striped bass lack specialized scales and are embedded in dermal bone where pores open directly from the canals through the integument to the environment.

A simple squamous epithelium lines the canal system except in the region adjacent to the neuromast cells, where it appears more cuboidal. The entire epithelial lining is continuous with that of the integument and may contain lymphocytes, coarse eosinophilic granular leukocytes, rodlet cells, and goblet cells that stain positively for acid mucosubstances. The neuromast is a bilayered receptor; its apical end consists of club shaped receptor cells, beneath which are located the basal nuclei of the sustentacular cells (Fig. 33C). The sustentacular cells extend processes up, between the sensory cells, to support its gelatinous matrix or cupula. Iwai (1967) suggested that the sustentacular cells secrete this matrix material. The cupula rests firmly upon the sensory hairs (kinocilia and steriocilia) that project out from the apical ends of the sensory cells (Flock 1967; Harder 1975) (see below). Both the epithelial lining of the canals and the neuromasts rest on a basement membrane, which is part of a vascular connective tissue sheath (Fig. 33C) that surrounds the canal and connects its epithelium to adjacent dermal bone and ossicles. In teleosts, according to Suckling (1967), the lateral-line nerve, innervating both canal and superficial neuromasts, contains branches of nerve twigs that ultimately connect wth the vagus or cranial nerve X in the trunk region and with cranial nerve VII in the head region.

In striped bass, superficial neuromasts occur primarily in the epidermis of the head and are structurally identical to but smaller than the canal neuromasts. Reno (1966) described two basic types of superficial teleost neuromasts, bell-shaped and onion-shaped (Fig. 33D), both of which occur perpendicular to the body surface in the striped bass (Fig. 33D,E). Although the cupulae were removed in this study during histological preparation, it generally is accepted that superficial neuromasts also bear cupulae (Hoar and Randall 1971).

The lateral-line canals are also believed to be filled with gelatinous or mucoid substances that hold the cupulae in place. The neuromasts, when stimulated by water movements, vibrate this mucoid matrix and bend the cupulae, causing excitation of sensory hairs (Grizzle and Rogers 1976). Although the precise acoustical function of the lateral-line system still is controversial, many authors believe that it perceives near-field pressure waves (Cahn 1966; Harder 1975; Tavolga 1976; Weber and Schiewe 1976), enabling the fish to seek out prey, ward off enemies, and avoid obstacles.

Stato-Acoustic Organ

The two stato-acoustic organs, or inner ears, of striped bass are histologically identical to those described for higher teleosts by Lowenstein (1971), Harder (1975), and Lagler et al. (1977). Unlike channel catfish (Grizzle and Rogers 1976) striped bass have no Weberian apparatus. Each ear is comprised of three semicircular canals (anterior, horizontal, and posterior) and three otolith chambers (utriculus, sacculus, and lagena) that are interconnected and filled with endolymph. The entire organ is contained in the cranial wall, being situated lateral and caudal to the medulla or ventral rhombencephalon of the brain (Figs. 26A, 34A).

The three semicircular canals are oriented perpendicular to one another and each has an ampulla located near its junction with the anterior otolith chamber or utriculus. Contained within the ampulla is the crista ampullaris, which histologically resembles the neuromasts of the lateral line system. Its macula contains elongated apical sensory cells with centrally placed nuclei and basal supporting cells, both of which are supported by a connective-tissue stalk (Fig. 34B). A cupula rests on top of these sensory cells and contacts sensory hairs (kinocilia and stereocilia) in just the same manner as those of the lateral-line system (Popper 1977). The canals are lined by a simple squamous epithelium, which is supported by and connected to the cranial bone by collagenous connective tissue, except proximal to the crista ampullaris where globular sensory epithelium can be distinguished (Fig. 34B).

The otolith chambers may contain large sensory areas or maculae that are flush with the chamber wall, and single calcified cupulae or otoliths (Fig. 34A) that are separated from one another by an otolith membrane. Popper (1977) stated that this membrane holds the otolith in place on top of the macula and thus provides a mechanical coupling between the otolith and the sensory hairs. The posterior two chambers, sacculus and lagena, extend caudad below the spinal cord near the foramen magnum in the striped bass. The anterior roots of the cranial nerve VIII innervate the utricular maculae and semicircular canal ampullae; the posterior roots of this nerve innervate the saccular and lagenar maculae.

The primary functions ascribed to the teleost stato-acoustic organs are those of balance and hearing. In particular, the semicircular canal ampulae help the fish perceive angular acceleration. This is accomplished when the canal endolymph pushes against the gelatinous cupulae to stimulate the sensory cells of the maculae. The otolith maculae are involved with sound reception and gravity perception. They transit body movement, sound vibration, and gravitational pull via the calcified cupulae or otoliths to the maculae, from which nerve impulses are passed to the brain (Harder 1975; Grizzle and Rogers 1976).

Olfactory Apparatus

The paired olfactory organs are in the nasal pits rostral to the eyes and consist of multiple lamellar folds oriented longitudinally along the inner wall of the nasal pits; the folds have an epithelial layer that is separated from the dermis by a prominent basement membrane (Fig. 34C).

Each nasal pit has two nostrils that allow water to pass freely over the chemosensory epithelium of the olfactory lamellae. Portions of this epithelium bear sensory endings that respond to chemical stimuli other than the four qualities—sweet, bitter, salty, and acid—that humans detect (Harder 1975). The axons of these primary sensory cells transit impulses directly to the brain via the olfactory or first cranial nerve (Kleerekoper 1969).

Yamamoto and Ueda (1977, 1978a, 1978b, 1978c, 1978d, 1978e, 1978f) described both sensory and nonsensory epithelium in the olfactory organs of several teleost families. Sensory epithelium is located along the lateral surfaces of the lamelar folds (Fig. 34D) in the striped bass olfactory organ. It contains bipolar neurons, sustentacular cells, nonsensory ciliated epithelial cells, basal cells, goblet cells, rodlet cells, lymphocytes, and eosinophilic glandular leukocytes (Bannister 1965; Harder 1975; Grizzle and Rogers 1976). The bipolar neurons or ganglionic cells of many teleosts have peripherally directed dendrites and extremely thin axons that join the olfactory bulb directly without an interconnecting neuron, according to Kleerekoper (1969). These unmyelinated axons join in the loose connective tissue of the submucosa to form the larger nerve bundles or fila of the olfactory nerve (Kreutzburg and Gross 1977) (Fig. 34E). In the striped bass, nonsensory epithelial cells (Fig. 34D) are best distinguished by their peripheral location, large circular nuclei, and cilia; in contrast, sensory neurons and sustentacular cells in the sensory epithelium have oval to elongated nuclei situated more basally. Intermingled among the sensory cells are goblet cells and rodlet cells, whereas basal cells, lymphocytes, and coarse eosinophilic granular leukocytes border the basal lamina and dermal olfactory elements.

A nonsensory epithelium covers the apical ends of the lamellar folds and the remaining surface of the nasal pit (Fig. 34F). It is stratified squamous along the tips of the lamellae and simple cuboidal to squamous elsewhere. Numerous goblet cells, rodlet cells, lymphocytes, and a few coarse eosinophilic granular leukocytes combine to form the more basal elements of this epithelium (Zeiske et al. 1976) (Fig. 34F).

Eye

Teleost eyes are bilateral sense organs that develop as outpocketings of the brain (Harder 1975). They are structurally similar to those found in all vertebrates (Fig. 35A), being situated in bony cavities or myodomes of the skull and attached to it by six striated oculomotor muscles and vascularized areolar connective tissue (conjunctiva). Each eye is integrated with the optic lobe of the brain via an optic nerve. In striped bass, the transparent cornea, which covers the external-lateral surface of the eye, has several layers of epithelial cells that are contiguous with the integument. Internally, the eye is surrounded by a cartilaginous sclera. Inside this lies the choroidea, containing an outer vascularized layer that supplies oxygen to the retina and an inner pigmented cell layer (choroid tapeta), which my function to reflect light transmitted through the retina to the vision cell layer (Zyznar 1975) (Fig. 35B). The iris is a continuation of the choroidea and extends out under the cornea. Adjacent to the inner layer of the choroidea is the retina, which is a ganglional extension of the mesencephalon. The optic nerves, the fibers of which originate in the retina, relay visual stimuli to the optic tectum. Located within the eye cavity between the aqueous and vitreous humor is the

---

Figure 34. Sensory organs of striped bass.

- **A.** Transverse section of the spinal cord and associated semicircular canals, 3-month-old fish (formalin; H&E). Bar = 209 μm.
- **B.** Crista in the ampulla of a semicircular canal, 3-month-old fish (Bouin's; H&E). Bar = 33 μm.
- **C.** Transverse section of the olfactory organ, 3-year-old fish (formol sublimate; HPS). Bar = 270 μm.
- **D.** Sensory olfactory epithelium, 3-year-old fish (formol sublimate; H&E). Bar = 9.2 μm.
- **E.** Nerve fibers in the olfactory lamellae, 3-year-old fish (formol sublimate; H&E). Bar = 23 μm.
- **F.** Nonsensory olfactory epithelium, 3-year-old fish (glutaraldehyde; TB). Bar = 9.6 μm.

1 Areolar connective tissue
2 Artery
3 Cranium
4 Crest of the olfactory lamellae
5 Crista ampullaris
6 Cupula
7 First cranial olfactory nerve bundles
8 Globular sensory cells of the ampullar epithelium
9 Goblet cells
10 Head kidney tissue
11 Lumen of the ampulla
12 Lymph vessel
13 Macula
14 Nonsensory ciliated epithelial cell
15 Olfactory lamellae
16 Olfactory mucosa
17 Otolith chamber (lagena)
18 Red blood cells
19 Rodlet cells
20 Semicircular canals (posterior)
21 Sensory cells
22 Skeletal muscle bundles
23 Spinal cord
24 Spinal ganglion
25 Submucosa of the lamellae
26 Sustentacular and receptor cell nuclei
27 Sustentacular cells (supporting cells)

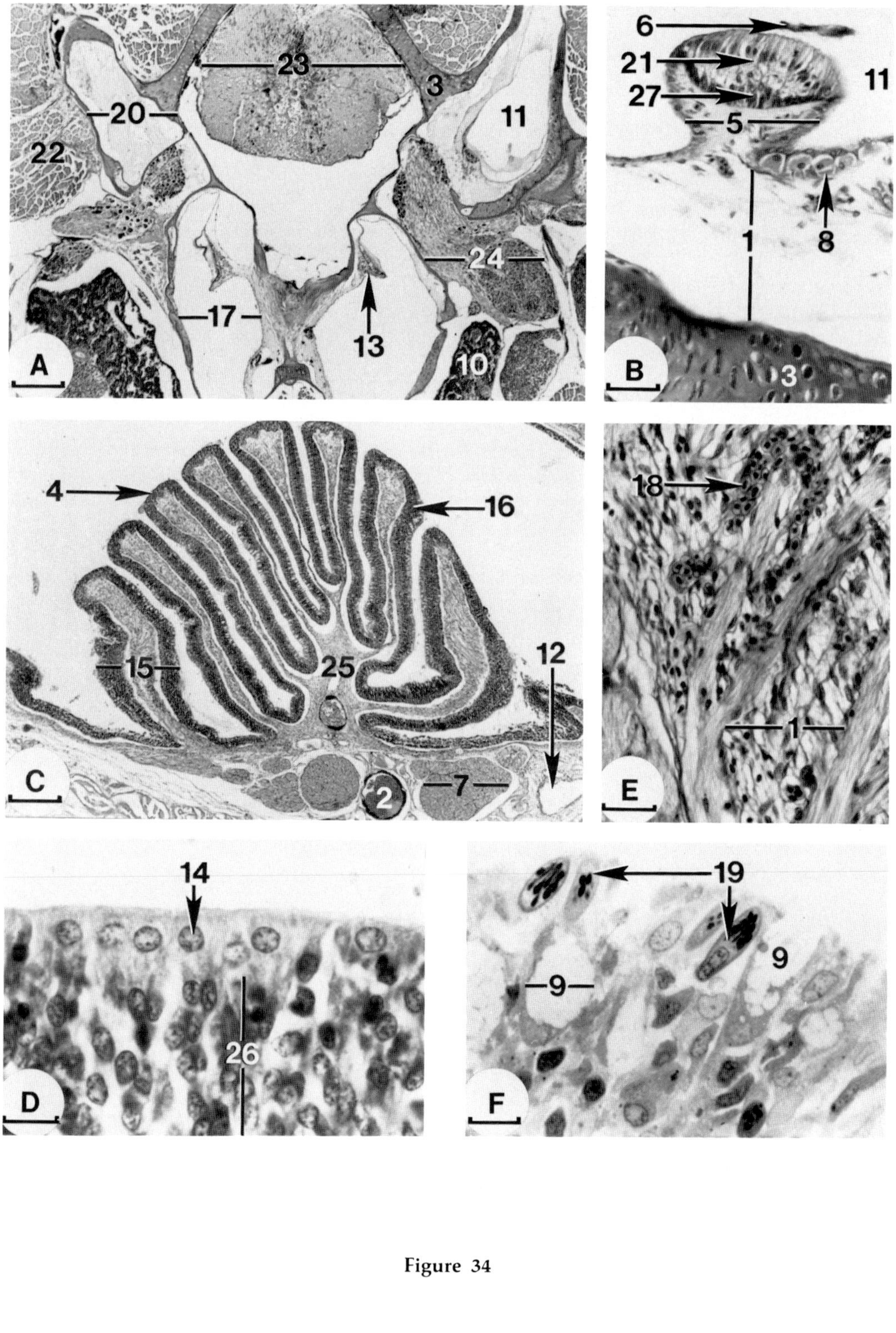
23
3
20
22
11
24
17
13
10
A
6
21
27
11
5
8
1
3
B
4
16
15
25
12
7
2
C
18
1
E
14
26
D
19
9
9
9
F

Figure 34

spherical lens consisting of crystalline fibers covered by a single epithelial layer. The lens is supported by the retractor lentis muscles and the suspensory ligaments, which move the lens back and forth to accommodate focusing (Harder 1975).

The comparative histology of teleost retinas has been thoroughly discussed by Harder (1975) and Ali and Anctil (1976). The retina of striped bass was studied by Faulkner (1952), who noted that its vision cells consist of rods, single cones, and double cones (Lyall 1957). All together, the ganglial components of the retina form nine distinct layers (Fig. 35C): outer epithelial layer; vision-cell layer; external limiting membrane; external nuclear layer; external plexiform layer; internal nuclear layer; internal plexiform layer; ganglion cell layer; and a nerve fiber layer that synapses wth the optic nerve. Visual images are relayed from the rods and cones of the vision layer to the nerve-fiber layer and then via the optic nerve to the mesencephalon for integration (Fig. 35D).

Of particular interest to teleost histologists is the choroid body within the chorioidea (Fig. 35B); it is present in fish like striped bass that possess pseudobranchiae. The choroid body is usually horseshoe-shaped and partially surrounds the entrance of the optic nerve into the eye. It forms an elaborate bipolar reté consisting of thousands of closely packed and parallel arterial mirabile and venous capillaries. The capillaries are arranged according to the counter-current principle like those of the gas bladder reté. Barnett (1951) theorized that the choriod body equalizes pressure differences inside and outside the eye. Beatty (1975) suggested that the reté, together with the pigment cell epithelium and choriocapillaries, maintains high oxygen tensions in the mainly avascular teleost retina. The exact function of this tissue, however, has yet to be resolved.

Figure 35. Eye of striped bass.

A. Transverse section of the eye (the break in the retina and detachment of the lens are artifacts), 3-month-old fish (formalin; HPS). Bar = 343 μm.
B. Choroideal tissue of an eye, 3-year-old fish (formalin; PTAH). Bar = 37 μm.
C. Retina of an eye, 3-year-old fish (formalin; HPS). Bar = 72 μm.
D. Optic nerve and retina, 3-month-old fish (formalin; H&E). Bar = 85 μm.

1 Blood vessels of the rete mirabile
2 Cartilagenous sclera
3 Choroidea and sclera
4 Cones
5 Cornea
6 Epithelial layer
7 External limiting membrane
8 External nuclear layer
9 External plexiform layer
10 Ganglion cell layer
11 Internal limiting membrane
12 Internal nuclear layer
13 Internal plexiform layer
14 Iris
15 Lens
16 Nerve fiber layer
17 Optic nerve
18 Pigment cells of the choroid tapeta
19 Retina
20 Rods
21 Visual cell layer

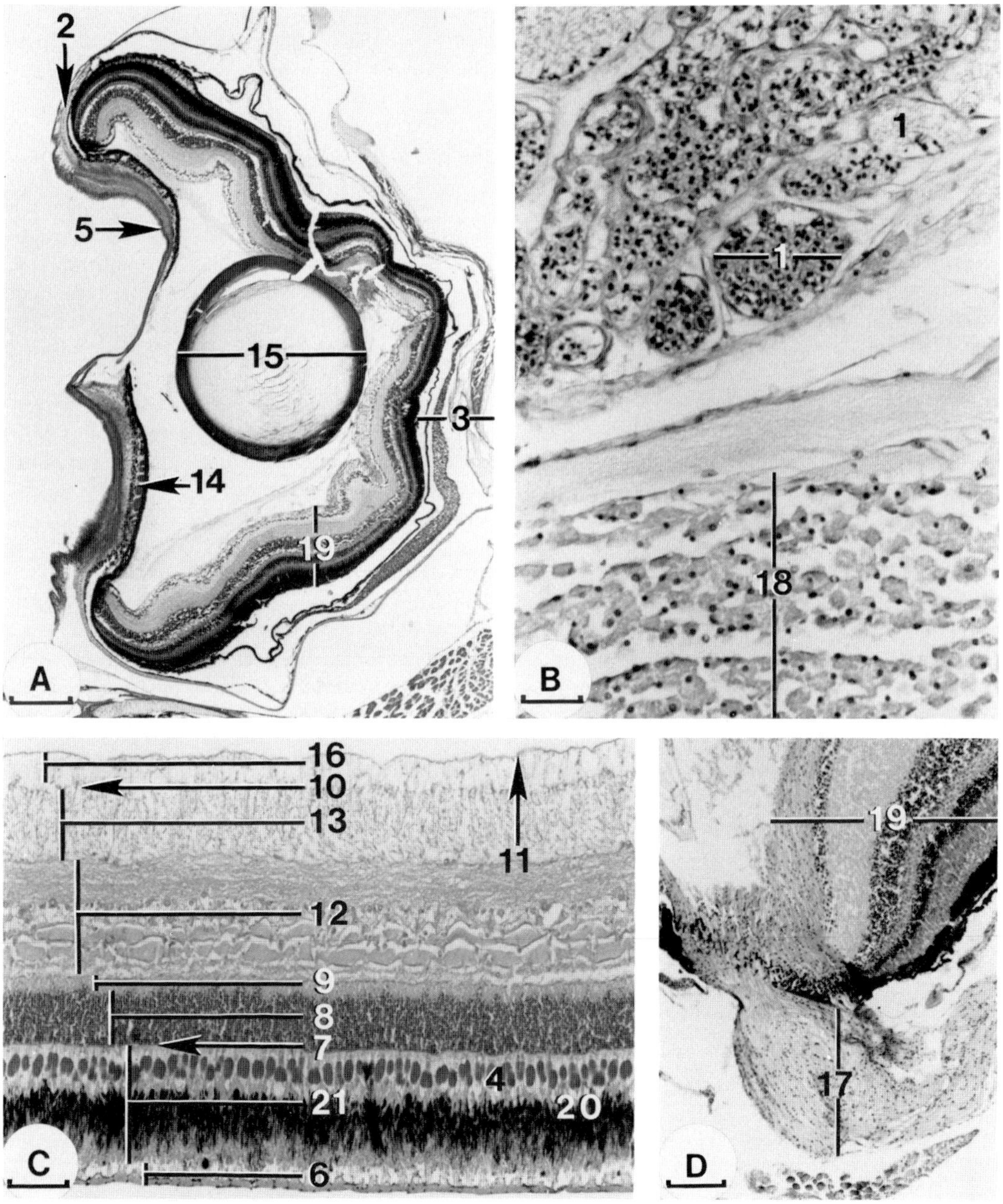

Figure 35

Endocrine System

Teleost endocrine tissues form ductless glands that are intimately associated with the vascular system, and usually are incorporated within other organs. At least fifteen tissues that possess endocrine activity occur in fish: pituitary; saccus vasculosus; pineal; urophysis; thyroid; ultimobranchial; thymus; pseudobranchiae; chromaffin tissue; interrenal tissue; corpuscles of Stannius; endocrine pancreas; enteroendocrine tissue of the gut; interstitial cells of the gonads; and the justaglomerular cells of the kidney (Harder 1975; Lagler et al. 1977). This study did not include histochemical identification of the latter three tissues. Descriptions of the saccus vasculosus and pineal organs are included with the Nervous System (page 72), the thymus with the Circulatory System (page 14), and the pseudobranchiae with the Respiratory System (page 46).

Pituitary Gland

The pituitary gland is suspended from the ventral hypothalamus of the diencephalon by a short infundibular stalk (Figs. 29A, 36A). It is composed of a neural element (neurohypophysis), formed by a downpocketing of the diencephalon, and an epithelial element (adenohypophysis), originating from the epithelium of the dorsal oral cavity (Ball and Baker 1969; Grizzle and Rogers 1976). These elements are separated from each other by a basement membrane or median eminence. This neuroendocrine gland is a major source of the hormones needed to coordinate and maintain physiological homeostasis in all fish.

According to Perks (1969), the basic elements of the teleost neurohypophysis include: secretory nuclei, that border the preoptic and infundibular recesses of the third ventricle (Fig. 36A); stainable Type-A_1 nerve fibers with 120-nm-diameter vesicles; Type-A_2 nerve fibers with 120-nm-diameter vesicles; nonstainable Type-B fibers with irregular 70-nm-diameter vesicles; glial cells (pituicytes); and blood vessels. The region of the neurohypophysis that interdigitates with the adenohypophysis is termed the pars nervosa (Fig. 36A,B). In striped bass, only pituicytes and secretory nuclei are evident in this tissue without the aid of special stains (Plate 4B). According to Perks (1969), fish neurosecretions originiating in the preoptic nuclei travel via Type-A_1 and -A_2 axons to the caudal pars nervosa, whereas neurosecretions originating in the lateral tuberal nuclei move down Type-B axons to the rostral pars nervosa. In mature fish, the stainable secretions often accumulate as Herring Bodies in the caudal pars nervosa

---

Figure 36. Endocrine glands of striped bass.

A. Sagittal section of the ventral hypothalamus (diencephalon), 3-month-old fish (formalin; H&E). Bar = 67 μm.
B. Transverse section of the pituitary (hypophysis), 3-year-old fish (Bouin–Allen's; H&E). Bar = 251 μm.
C. Dorsal region of the urophysis, 3-year-old fish (Helly's; H&E). Bar = 74 μm.
D. Transverse section of the tongue, 3-month-old fish (formalin; H&E). Bar = 87 μm.
E. Thyroid follicles, 3-year-old fish (Bouin's; H&E). Bar = 21 μm.

1 Areolar connective tissue
2 Capillary
3 Cranium
4 Cuboidal epithelial cells
5 Follicular colloid
6 Infundibular recess
7 Jugular vein
8 Medial lobe of the hypothalamus
9 Mixed bone
10 Musculus geniohyoideus (genihyoid muscle)
11 Nerve fibers of medulla
12 Neurohypophysial strands
13 Neurosecretory cells
14 Oral cavity
15 Oral mucosa
16 Pars intermedia
17 Periventricular hypothalamic region
18 Pituitary (hypophysis)
19 Proximal pars distalis
20 Red blood cells
21 Rostral pars distalis
22 Saccus vasculosus
23 Taste buds
24 Thyroid follicles
25 Ventral aorta

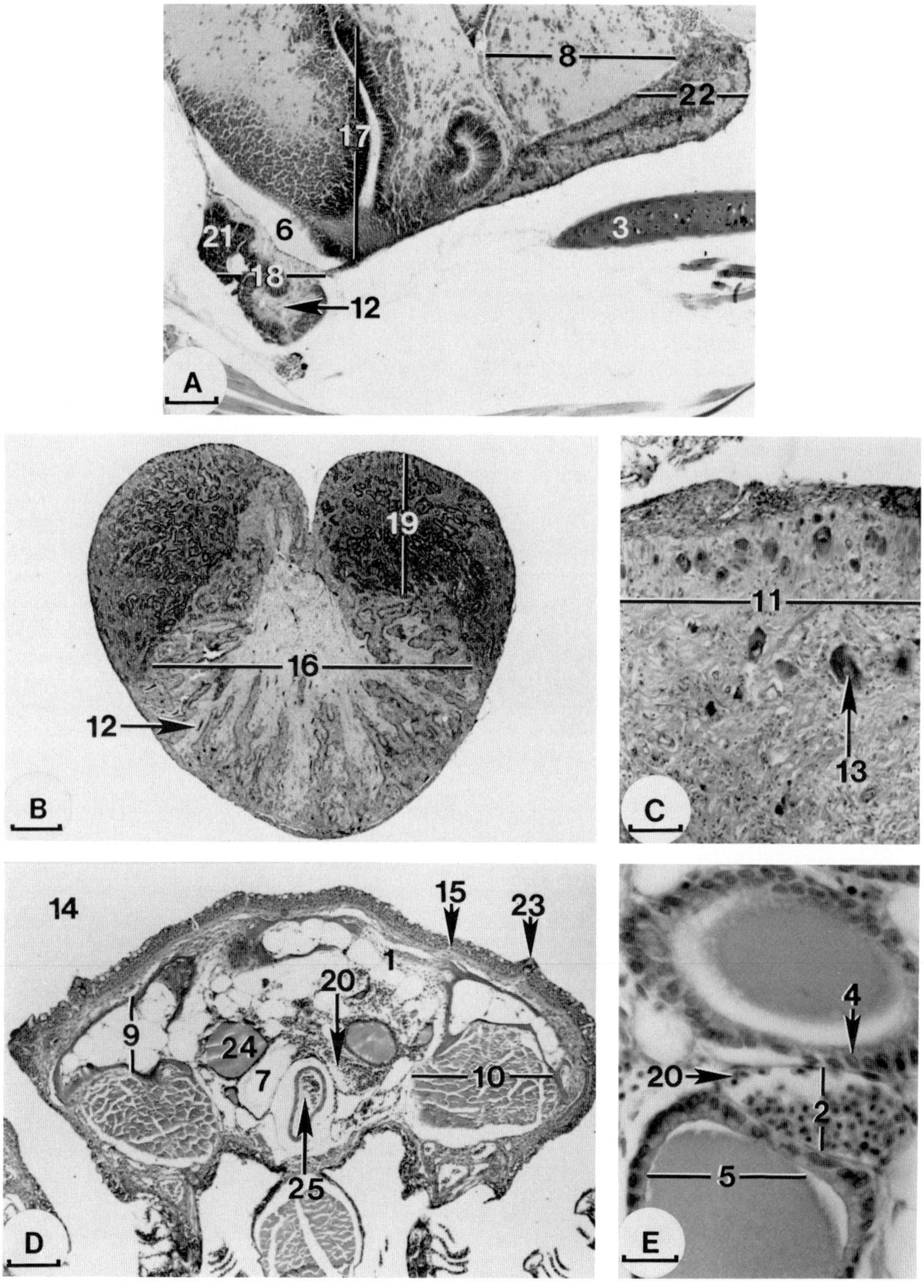
8
22
17
3
21
6
18
12
A
19
16
12
B
11
13
C
14
15
23
1
20
9
24
7
10
25
D
4
20
2
5
E

Figure 36

(Perks 1969; Anderson and Mitchum 1974). Control of the adenohypophysis, osmoregulation, and reproduction have been attributed to the neurohypophysis in higher teleosts (Hoar and Randall 1969).

The adenohypophysis of the striped bass has three histologically distinct regions: rostral pars distalis; caudal or proximal pars distalis; pars intermedia (Fig. 36A,B). These designations are based upon tinctorial responses of the pituitary epithelium to various staining techniques applied in this study (Table 3) (Gabe 1976).

Rostral Pars Distalis

The rostral pars distalis lies in the most anterior and dorsal regions of adenohypophysis. Three cell types can be identified in this area. Type-I cells, which occupy most of the rostral pars distalis, stain orange with the Azan technique, are rounded, and have eccentrically placed kidney-shaped nuclei (Plate 3D,E). Recent literature (Ball and Baker 1969; Boddingius 1975; Jose and Sathyanesan 1977) strongly suggests that these are the prolactin cells of the teleost pituitary. Follicles of prolactin cells, such as those found in rainbow trout and other isopondylous species, are not present in striped bass (Ball and Baker 1969). Type-II cells are arranged in islands toward the periphery of the rostral pars distalis and their cytoplasm stains dark blue-purple by the aldehyde fuchsin Halmi (AFH) method and blue-green with the Azan technique (Plate 3E). These cells appear angular or polymorphic in shape, contain rounded nuclei, and are believed to be gonadotrophs (Ball and Baker 1969; Schreibman et al. 1973; Jose and Sathyanesan 1977). Type-III cells are located in a band perpendicular to the rostral pars nervosa (Plate 3D). These chromophobic cells stain light orange with the Azan method, appear cylindrical or club-shaped, and contain oval or rounded nuclei. Much controversy surrounds their function as some authors consider them corticotrophs (Ball and Baker 1969; Schreibman et al. 1973), that are involved in the production of ACTH (adrenocorticotropic hormone), whereas others (Boddingius 1975) indicate that much of the supportive experimental evidence for this function is conflicting.

Caudal Pars Distalis

The caudal pars distalis is ventral to the rostral pars nervosa and lateral to the dorsal pars intermedia. It is the most vascularized region of the pituitary and contains four distinct cell types. Type-IV cells are arranged in cords that border both the ventrally penetrating elements and the blood vessels of the pars nervosa (Plate 3F). These cells appear histologically similar to Type-I cells but stain red-orange with the Azan technique. The literature (Ball and Baker 1969; Jose and Sathyanesan 1977) indicates that they may function as

Table 3. *Tinctorial properties of pituitary cells from a 3-year-old female striped bass sampled during July and fixed in Helly's fluid.*

Location	Cell type	Probable functional equivalent	Stain and color		
			CHP[a]	AFH[b]	AZAN[c]
Rostral pars distalis	I	Prolactin cells (acidophilic)	Pink		Orange
	II	Gonadotrophs (granulated and strongly basophilic)	Blue-black	Purple	Blue-green
	III	Corticotrophs (chromophobic)	Light pink		Light pink
Caudal par distalis	IV	Somatotrophs (acidophilic)	Dark pink		Red-orange
	V	Thryotrophs (lightly basophilic)	Blue-black	Purple	Blue-green
	VI	Inactive gonadotrophs (chromophobic)	Light pink		Orange
	II	Gonadotrophs (granulated and strongly basophilic)	Blue-black	Purple	Blue-green
Pars intermedia	VII	Unknown function (acidophilic)	Pink		Orange
	VIII	Melanocyte stimulating hormone? (chromophobic)	Light pink	Light purple	Grey-green
	IX	Gonadotrophs (degranulated and lightly basophilic)	Blue-black	Purple	Light blue-green
	II	Gonadotrophs (granulated and strongly basophilic)	Blue-black	Purple	Blue-green

[a] Chrome-hematoxylin phloxine (Gabe 1976).
[b] Aldehyde fuchsin, Halmi (Gabe 1976).
[c] Azocarmine B and aniline blue, Mallory–Heidenhain (Gabe 1976).

somatotrophs. In striped bass, Type-V cells are scattered in the dorsal region of the caudal pars distalis or between cords of Type-IV cells (Plate 3F) and have an angular morphology, a rounded nucleus, and a lightly basophilic cytoplasm (Table 3). The tinctorial characteristics and morphologic location indicate that they may function as thyrotrophs, even though much of the staining of striped bass material was indistinct and no definitive characterization could be made (Ball and Baker 1969). Chromophobic Type-VI cells have oval to rounded nuclei and extremely little cytoplasm and stain faintly orange by the Azan technique. They are located throughout the adenohypophysis, with the largest population occurring in the ventral region of the caudal pars distalis, which suggests that they may represent inactive gonadotrophs in post-spawning striped bass (Schreibman et al. 1973). Basophilic Type-II cells also were present in the ventral region of the caudal pars distalis and along its junction with the pars intermedia.

Pars Intermedia

The pars intermedia occupies nearly one-half of the striped bass pituitary (Fig. 36B) and is penetrated by more neurohypophyseal fibers than any other region of the gland. Together with the caudal pars nervosa, it forms a wedge of tissue that fans out caudoventrally from the dorsal pituitary stalk. Four cell types are present in this region (Table 3). Type-VII cells are oval and occupy a single layer perpendicular to the neurohypophysial strands (Plate 4A). These cells have oval or compressed nuclei and cytoplasm that stains orange by the Azan technique and pink with the chrome-hematoxylin phloxine (CHP) method. Again, much confusion surrounds the hormonal function of this cell; Boddingius (1975) suggested an MSH (melanophore-stimulating hormone) function, but other authors (Ball and Baker 1969; Schreibman et al. 1973) present conflicting support for this hormone and even suggest an osmoregulatory function. No definitive statement can be made for the striped bass, because only MSH has been positively identified as a product of the pars intermedia in teleosts (Ball and Baker 1969). Type-VII cells are arranged toward the interior of the pars intermedia strands (Plate 4A,B). These polygonal cells contain rounded nuclei and elongated cytoplasmic processes, which often contact interdigitating neurohypophysial strands. The cytoplasm stains grey-green by the Azan technique and a light pink with the CHP method. Bright red inclusions are present in their cytoplasm, suggesting hormonal accumulations or degenerative cellular components (Boddingius 1975) (Plate 4B). Most of the literature (Ball and Baker 1969; Schreibman et al. 1973) agrees that MSH production can positively be attributed to Type-VIII cells. Type-IX cells most often are found in close proximity to Type-II gonadotrophs along the ventral pituitary and occasionally at the periphery of pars intermedia strands (Plate 4A). The former cell type appears degranulated, stains lightly basophilic (Table 3), has a rounded nucleus and a polygonal shape, and is larger than the Type-II gonadotrophs. Type-IX cells should be considered degranulated gonadotrophs (Ball and Baker 1969; Schreibman et al. 1973; Boddingius 1975).

Caudal Neurosecretory System

The primary element of the caudal neurosecretory system is the urophysis spinalis, an oval stalked ventral appendage of the spinal cord. It is embedded within a depression termed the urostylar fossa, which is formed between the preterminal vertebra and the urostyle of the backbone (Jaiswol and Belsare 1973). The urophysis spinalis is well vascularized by elements of the caudal aorta and caudal vein, through which its urotensil hormones are dispersed readily into the blood stream (Harder 1975; Grizzle and Rogers 1976). This endocrine organ shares histological elements with the caudal spinal cord, such as neurosecretory Dahlgren cells, glial and ependymal cells, nerve fibers, numerous blood capillaries, and connective-tissue elements of the meninx primitiva and leptomeninx. The urophysis spinalis has a darker-staining, more vascularized cortex bearing neurosecretory products, and a more cellular medulla containing neurosecretory cells (Fig. 36C, Plate 4C). The caudal spinal cord contains most of the Dahlgren cell bodies, although some are present in the proximal medullary region of the urophysis. These polyhedral multinucleate giant cells bear several nerve processes that extend ventrally into the urophysis spinalis from the spinal cord. Capillary processes often are seen in close proximity to the Dahlgren cells and may even penetrate them, according to Jaiswol and Belsare (1973). Staining of the urophysis by the azorarmine-B and aniline-blue technique and with crystal violet and aldehyde fuchsin, readily depicted acidophilic colloidal droplets of neurosecretory material (Plate 4D), the multinucleated Dahlgren cells (Plate 4E), and the stored neurosecretory products of the cortex (Plate 4C) (Bern and Takasugi 1962).

Berlind (1973) and Chevalier (1978) suggested that four urotensins are produced by the urophysis spinalis, each of which has a specific hormonal function. Urotensin-I seems to influence blood pressure in fish, urotensin-II affects smooth muscle activity, urotensin-III helps to regulate sodium-ion movements, and urotensin-IV is thought to be involved with hydrosomatic activation. Berlind and Chevalier also suggested that these hormones may influence other hydromineral balances, as well as reproduction, osmoregulation, and kidney function in teleosts.

Thyroid Organ

The thyroid organ is composed of unencapsulated follicles scattered diffusely along the dorsal and lateral aspects of the jugular veins and ventral aorta in striped bass (Fig. 36D). These follicles have colloid-filled lumens that are surrounded by an expandable glandular epithelium, which may appear either cuboidal or squamous depending upon the activity of the organ. This eosinophilic colloid comprises the reserve of potential hormone for the thyroid, which is the only vertebrate endocrine organ with such an extracellular store (Sage 1973). The loose connective tissue that surrounds the follicles is highly vascularized, having both anastomosing capillaries and lymph sinuses (Harder 1975). In most instances, the basally located nuclei of the follicular cells contact the endothelial lining of these capillaries (Fig. 36E).

The thyroid functions in the accumulation of iodine and the formation of thyroxin (Anderson and Mitchum 1974), which occurs in two forms: tetraiodothyronine and triiodothyronine. These hormones influence numerous metabolic processes, such as growth, differentiation, metamorphosis, maturation, reproduction, integumental development, respiration, migratory behavior, central nervous system activity, seasonal adaptations, temperature tolerance, osmoregulation, and possibly others (Sage 1973; Honma et al. 1977; Schreck and Scanlon 1977).

Endocrine Pancreas

The endocrine pancreas or islets of Langerhans are located amid exocrine pancreatic tissue along the mesenteries connecting the gall bladder and liver in striped bass. As noted in the section on extramural glands, this endocrine tissue forms true Brockman bodies as defined by Brinn (1973) (Fig. 37A,B). The large islets of endocrine tissue exhibit a true capsule, which also may encompass varying amounts of exocrine pancreatic tissue (Epple and Lewis 1973) (Fig. 37A). Within the islets, exocrine acini are separated by only a single connective tissue cell from the endocrine tissue (Plate 4F,G).

The cellular components of the islets are of particular interest as both the insulin and the glucagon produced by them are extremely important regulators of carbohydrate metabolism. The beta cells, which produce insulin, are located more centrally within the islets and can be distinguished easily by their smaller cytoplasmic granules, angular morphology, eccentric nucleus, and affinity for aldehyde fuchsin (Epple 1967) (Plate 4F). Alpha cells, which produce glucagon, are identified by the affinity of their larger granules for phosphotungstic acid hematoxylin (Levene and Feng 1964), peripheral position in the islets, larger oval morphology, rounded nucleus, and distinct eccentric nucleolus (Plate 4G). Although delta cells, amphi-

Figure 37. Endocrine glands of a 3-year-old striped bass.

A. The pancreas (formalin; HPS). Bar = 253 μm.
B. Pancreatic tissue (Helly's; PTAH). Bar = 38 μm.
C. Transverse section of the trunk kidney (formalin; H& E). Bar = 188 μm.
D. Corpuscle of Stannius (formalin; H&E). Bar = 37 μm.
E. Hematopoietic and mixed adrenal tissue of the head kidney (Bouin's; HPS). Bar = 80 μm.
F. Interrenal tissue (formalin; H&E). Bar = 9.5 μm.

1 Acellular bone
2 Acini of exocrine pancreas
3 Capsule of pancreatic islet
4 Columnar glandular epithelium of interrenal gland
5 Cords of corpuscle cells
6 Corpuscle of Stannius
7 Ductus choledochus
8 Endocrine pancreatic tissue
9 Endothelium
10 Hematopoietic tissue
11 Kidney tubules
12 Mixed adrenal tissue (interrenal and chromaffin)
13 Opisthonephric ducts
14 Pancreatic islet (endocrine and exocrine tissue)
15 Posterior cardinal vein
16 Red blood cells
17 Sinusoids of posterior cardinal vein
18 Skeletal muscle
19 Sympathetic ganglion
20 Zymogen granules

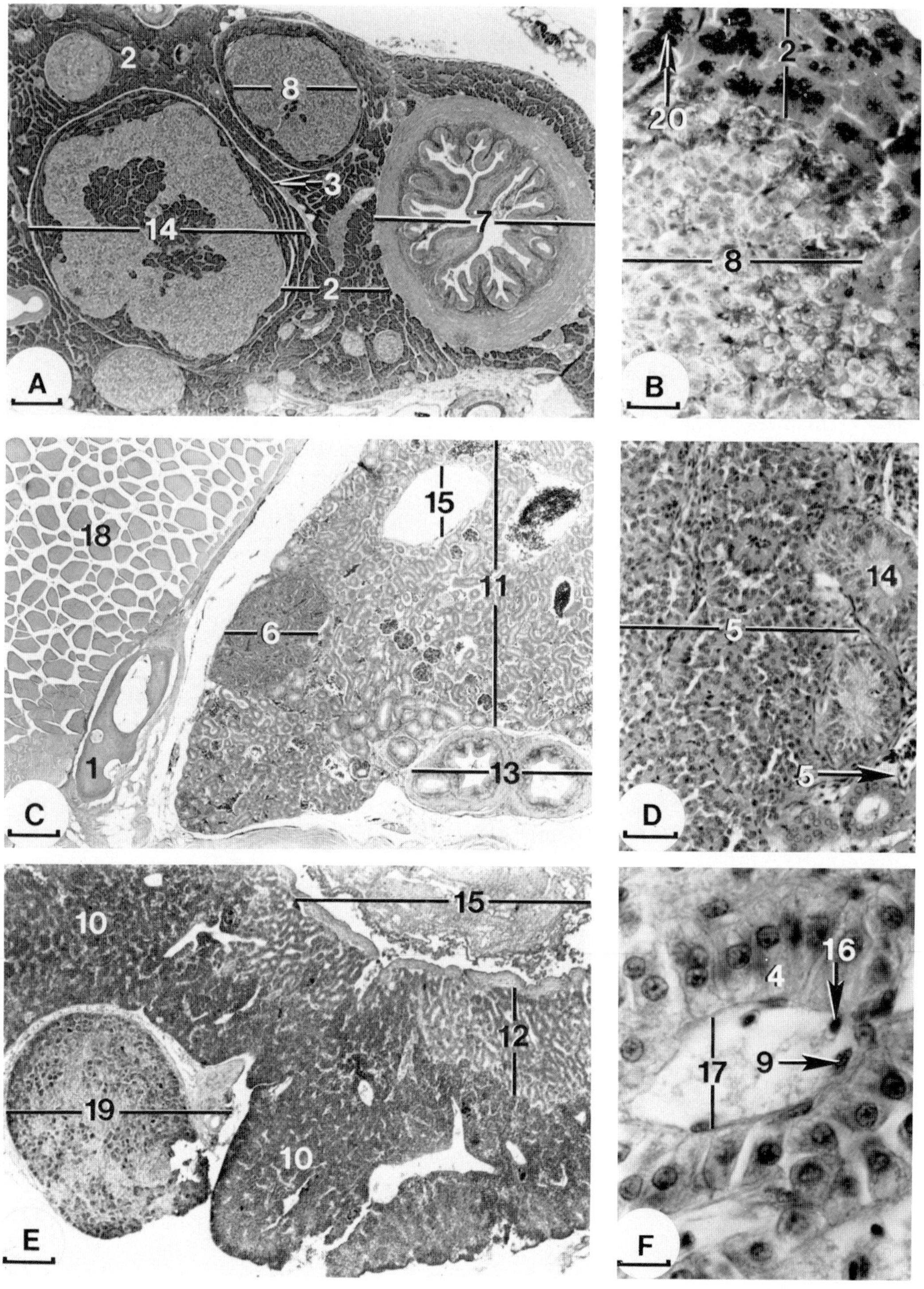

Figure 37

phils, and X-cells all have been reported in other teleosts, these islet components could not be identified by the staining methods employed in this study (Epple and Lewis 1973). Johnson et al. (1976) have suggested that somatostatin is the third hormone produced by delta cells in channel catfish. Similarly, Klein (1977) stated that these cells produce somatostatin or gastrin-like substances. However, evidence for the role of delta cells in the regulation of insulin and glucagon metabolism needs further confirmation.

Corpuscles of Stannius

Two discrete corpuscles of Stannius are present in striped bass. They are located on both ventrolateral walls of the trunk kidney approximately two-thirds of its length caudad (Fig. 37C). Unlike those of trout (Anderson and Mitchum 1974), these corpuscles are not visible along the peritoneal surface of the striped bass trunk kidney; rather, they are located deep within the kidney and are enclosed by a thin connective-tissue capsule that separates them from renal tubular elements. The corpuscles contain anastomosing bilaminar cords composed of short columnar to oval epithelium with basal nuclei. The cords are covered by a thin basal lamina and are separated from each other by connective tissue, as described for the threespine stickleback by Bonga et al. (1977). The apical cytoplasm of the glandular cells adjoins capillaries that penetrate the connective tissue septa; the nuclei of these cells abut one another toward the interior of the bilaminar cords (Fig. 37D). The portal system of the Stannius corpuscles receives blood from the dorsal caudal vein and the veins of the hypaxial musculature and is drained by veins that enter the caudal portion of the trunk kidney. In other teleosts like the threespine stickleback, the corpuscles are penetrated, along the vascular sinuses, by sympathetic nerves originating from the subvertebral ganglia (Belsare 1973; Bonga et al. 1977). In addition, Unsicker et al. (1977) suggested that chromaffin cells occur in the corpuscles of trout. Although nerve fibers are present in striped bass corpuscles, no histochemical confirmation of their origin was completed and no chromaffin cells were observed.

In anadromous species such as American eel, two cell types are commonly reported as constituents of the corpuscular cords: oval Type-1 cells, which tend to predominate, and slender Type-2 cells. Only Type-1 cells are thought to produce a hypocalciemic factor or hypocalcin. Youson and Butler (1976) suggested that this factor may help lower blood calcium concentrations and is more actively produced when a fish enters seawater. Type-2 cells are believed to be involved with the control of monovalent ions such as chlorine, sodium, and potassium (Borga et al. 1976, 1977; Olivereau and Olivereau 1978). Unsicker et al. (1977) contend that production, storage, or release of corpuscle hormones is mediated by monoamines in nerves and chromaffin cells of this organ. In addition to calcium regulation, Grizzle and Rogers (1976) suggested that the corpuscles of Stannius may function in osmoregulation, steroid production or storage, and renin production.

Interrenal Tissue

The interrenal tissue of fish is considered the homologue of the adrenal cortex in mammals (Anderson and Mitchum 1974). In striped bass, this unencapsulated endocrine organ is located in pockets adjoining the posterior cardinal veins in the head kidney (Fig. 37E). It is composed of anastomosing cords, usually bilaminar, of cuboidal or columnar epithelium with large central nuclei (Figs. 37F, 38A). These cells stain acidophilic

Figure 38. Endocrine glands of a 3-year-old striped bass.

A. Mixed adrenal tissue in wall of cardinal vein (formalin; H&E). Bar = 44 μm.
B. Chromaffin tissue along a vein in the trunk kidney (formalin; H&E). Bar = 26 μm.
C. Chromaffin tissue in the wall of the posterior cardinal vein (formalin; H&E). Bar = 24 μm.
D. Transverse section and the ultimobranchial body (formalin; H&E). Bar = 44 μm.
E. Ultimobranchial epithelium (formalin; PTAH). Bar = 16 μm.

1 Areolar connective tissue
2 Capillaries
3 Chromaffin cells
4 Columnar glandular epithelium
5 Dense connective tissue
6 First proximal kidney tubule
7 Interrenal tissue
8 Lumen of the ultimobranchial cyst
9 Nerve fibers
10 Posterior cardinal vein
11 Red blood cells
12 Second proximal kidney tubule
13 Sinusoids of posterior cardinal vein
14 Ultimobranchial body
15 Wall of the posterior cardinal vein

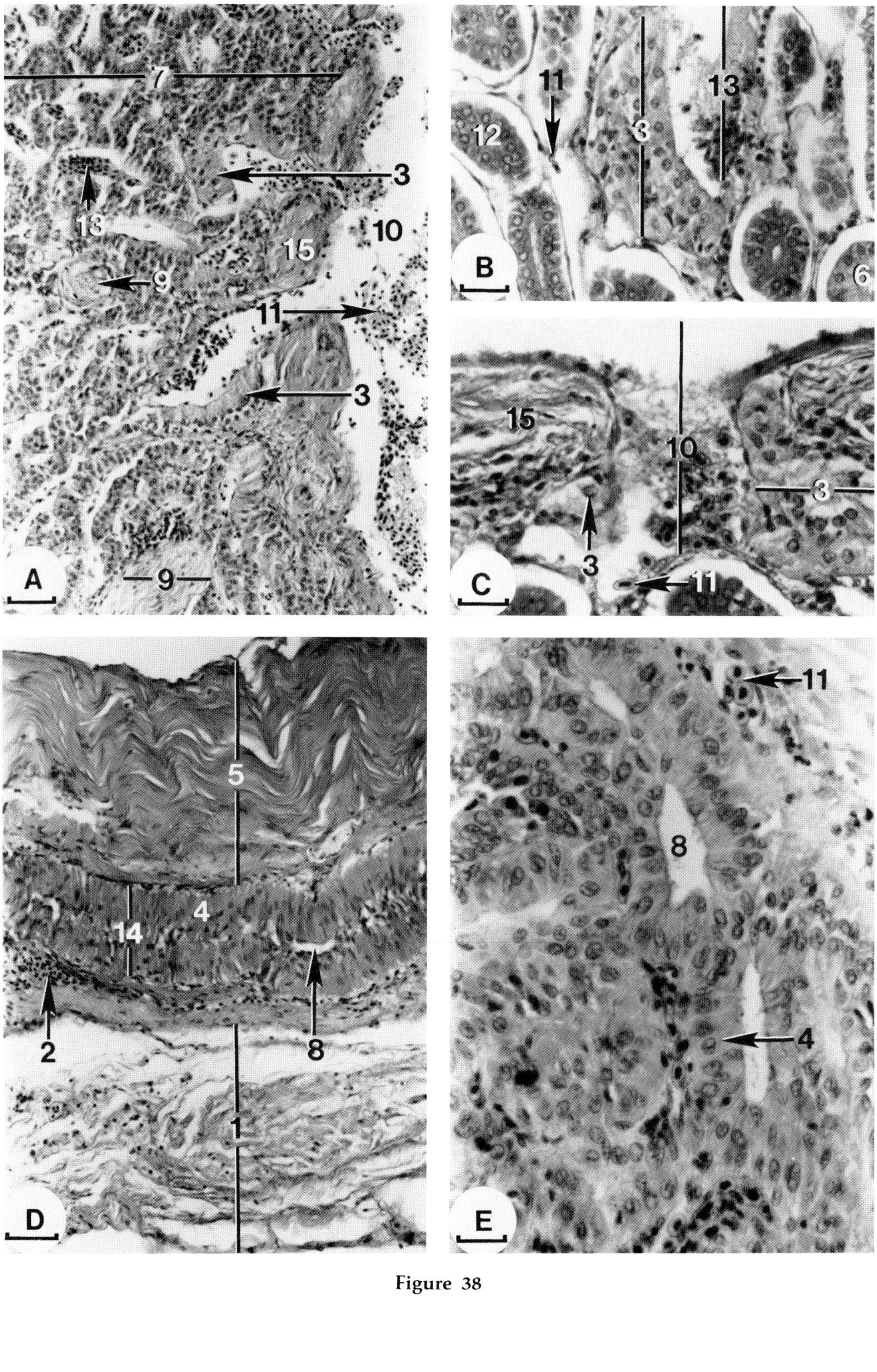

Figure 38

in comparison to the surrounding lymphomyeloid tissue. The cords are penetrated by nerve fibers and blood sinuses or tributaries of the posterior cardinal vein the endothelium of which contacts the apical cytoplasm of the interrenal cells (Fig. 37F) (Harder 1975; Youson et al. 1976). This type of cord structure agrees with the Type-I interrenal tissue classification of Nandi (1962).

The teleost interrenal tissue supplies glucocorticoids (cortisol, cortisone, corticosterone, and aldosterone) to the blood stream, and thus plays a major role in carbohydrate metabolism (Anderson and Mitchum 1974; Grizzle and Rogers 1976). The steroids it produces also may influence osmoregulation, hyponatremia, active transport, general stress response, blood cell maintenance, protein metabolism, reproduction, and spawning behavior (Schreck and Scanlon 1977). Control over interrenal function has been attributed to acetylcholine metabolism in the pituitary (Dixit 1970; Harder 1975).

Chromaffin Tissue

The chromaffin tissue of teleosts is considered homologous to the adrenal medulla of mammals (Anderson and Mitchum 1974). It occurs just under the endothelium or within the wall of the posterior cardinal veins and their tributaries throughout the kidney (Fig. 38A,B,C). This tissue is composed of pale-staining, irregularly shaped epithelial cells with large, rounded, central nuclei (Fig. 38B,C). In striped bass, chromaffin cells are located adjacent to cords of interrenal tissue or as isolated clumps along the capillary branches of the posterior cardinal vein in the trunk kidney (Fig. 38B) (Dixit 1970; Butler 1973). This arrangement fits the Type-IV chromaffin tissue classification of Nandi (1962), and resembles the distribution noted in the fathead minnow by Yoakim and Grizzle (1980).

Teleost chromaffin tissue originates from nerve ganglia (Fig. 37E) and produces adrenalin and noradrenalin. These two sympathomimetic hormones have systemic activity that is released instantaneously by stress (Grizzle and Rogers 1976; Schreck and Scanlon 1977). Presumably, two distinct cell types are responsible for the production of these hormones in fish (Anderson and Mitchum 1974). Youson (1976) noted only one cell type in bowfin electron microscopy, whereas Yoakim and Grizzle (1980) described two cell types in the fathead minnow. Only one cell type could be distinguished by light microscopy in the striped bass, although no attempt was made histochemically to identify these cells.

Ultimobranchial Organ

The calcium-regulating ultimobranchial organ is within the transverse septum separating the peritoneal cavity from the pericardial cavity. In striped bass, it resides dorsal to the insertion of the hepatic vein to the sinus venosus and ventral to the esophageal wall (Figs. 3B, 38D). In most teleosts, the ultimobranchial bodies are paired (Harder 1975, Grizzle and Rogers 1976). This may be true for striped bass as well; however, I could not confirm the presence of two distinct bodies.

The striped bass ultimobranchial organ is composed of ductless cavities lined by a columnar epithelium that forms both simple follicular structures or cysts and secondary follicles similar to those reported in rainbow trout and cherry salmon (McMillan et al. 1976; Yamane and Yamada 1977) (Fig. 38D,E). Dense connective tissue borders this organ on the peritoneal side of the septum; looser connective tissue borders it on the pericardial side. A capillary network, which connects directly with the sinus venosus, is intimately associated with the columnar epithelium (Fig. 38E). Harder (1975) stated that two cell types, oval barrel-shaped cells and slender finger cells, make up the glandular epithelium, which is the source of the calcitonin produced by the teleost ultimobranchial organ. Zaccone (1977) distinguished the two cell types as being either light- or dark-staining; Yamane and Yamada (1977) suggested that these cells are homologous with parafollicular "C" cells of the thyroid gland in mammals. McMillan et al. (1976) confirmed that the calcitonin is located primarily within the glandular epithelium of rainbow trout and not the cyst of the organ, though desquamated epithelial cells may be found here. In striped bass, the ultimobranchial epithelium may appear pseudostratified (Fig. 38D) or simple (Fig. 38E), but oval or barrel-shaped cells with basal nuclei predominate.

Calcitonin maintains hypocalcemic serum by opposing the resorption of bone by osteoclasts (Harder 1975). Its role in teleost metabolism is confusing. Bently (1976) noted that calcitonin has no effect on acellular bone of marine fish, but does effect freshwater fish with cellular bone. Thus, its hypocalcemic effect would be active in teleost bone that displays osteocytic and osteoclastic activity, such as in striped bass and other anadromous species. Pang (1971) noted that the gonads, corpuscles of Stannius, thyroid, interrenal, and pineal tissues all may be involved in calcium metabolism as well. An additional role in osmoregulation has also been suggested for calcitonin (Grizzle and Rogers 1976).

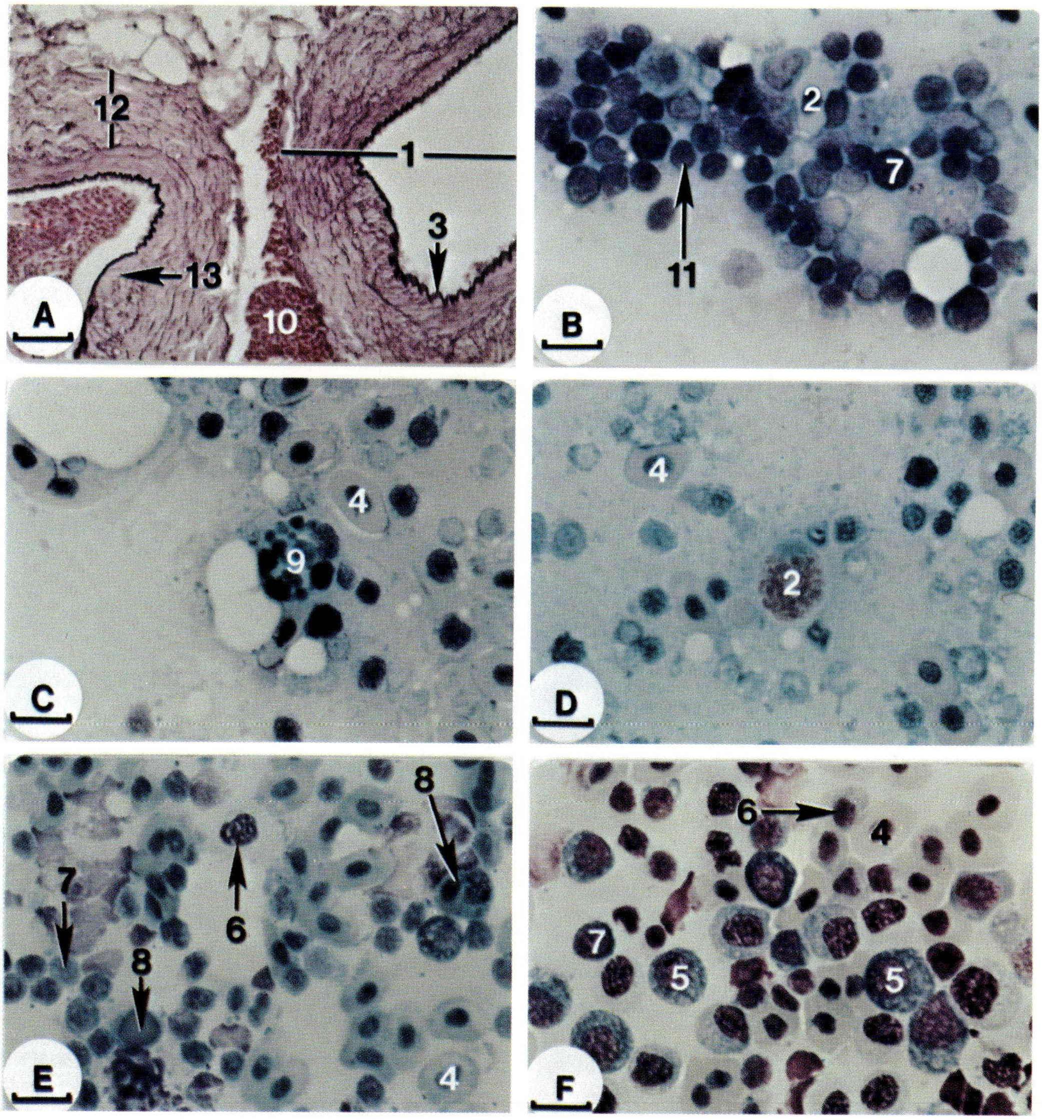

Plate 1. Circulatory and hematopoietic tissues of a 3-year-old striped bass.

A. Transverse section of a mesenteric artery (Helly's; AFH). Bar = 61 μm.
B. Thymus impression (methanol; Giemsa). Bar = 10 μm.
C. Tissue impression of the thymus, basophilic macrophage (methanol; Giemsa). Bar = 10 μm.
D. Tissue impression of the thymus, coarse eosinophilic granular leukocyte (methanol; Giemsa). Bar = 10 μm.
E. Spleen impression (methanol; Giemsa). Bar = 10 μm.
F. Head kidney impression (methanol; Giemsa). Bar = 10 μm.

1 Artery
2 Coarse eosinophilic granular leukocyte
3 Elastic membrane of the tunica intima
4 Erythrocyte (red blood cell)
5 Hemoblasts
6 Immature erythrocyte (reticulocyte)
7 Lymphocyte (small)
8 Macrophage with engulfed erythrocyte
9 Macrophage with basophilic inclusions
10 Red blood cells in a vein
11 Thymocyte
12 Tunica adventitia
13 Tunica media

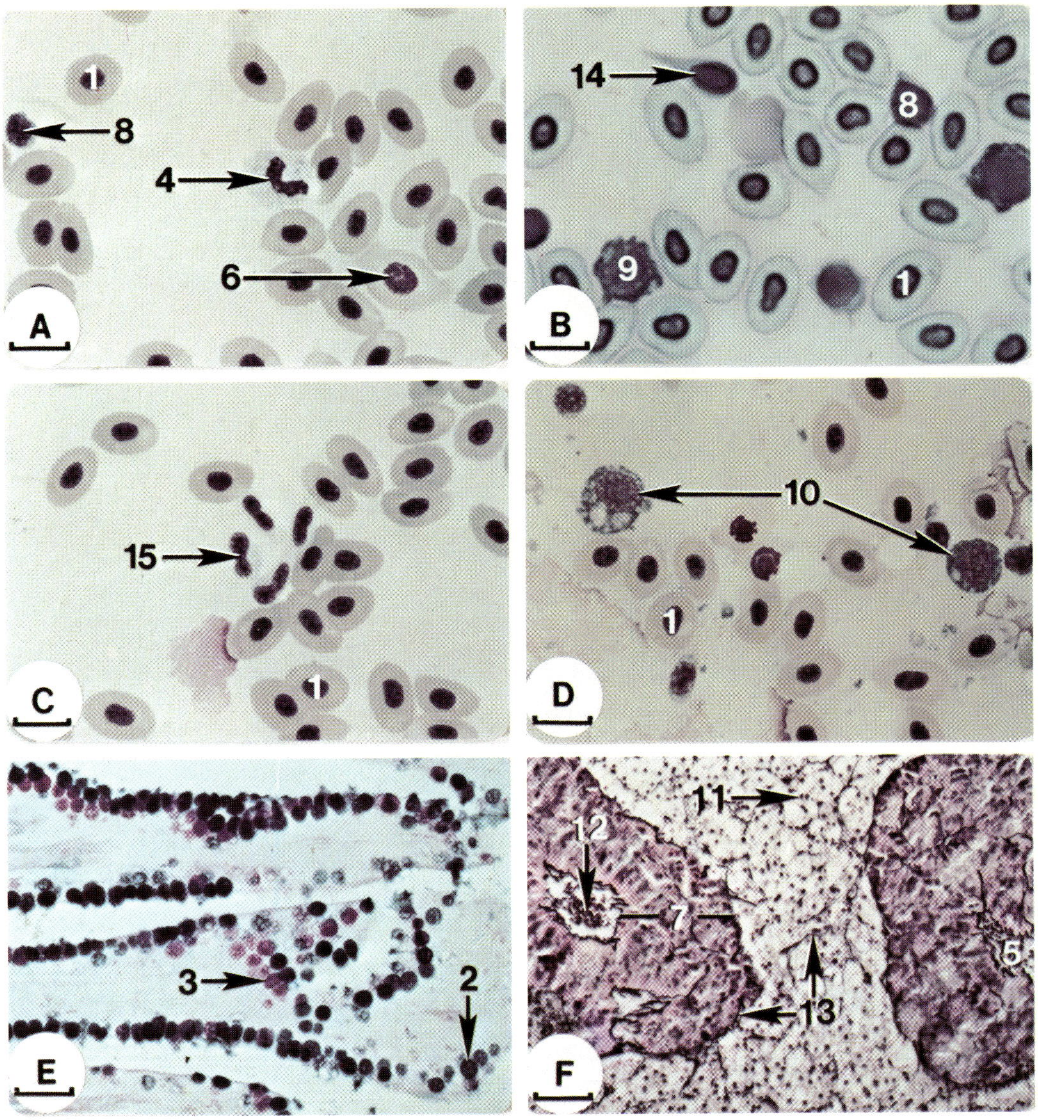

Plate 2. Blood and digestive-system tissues of a 3-year-old striped bass.

A. Blood film of erythrocytes and a granulocyte (methanol; Giemsa). Bar = 10 μm.
B. Blood film of erythrocytes, lymphocytes, and thrombocytes (methanol; Wright's). Bar = 10 μm.
C. Blood film of erythrocytes and thrombocytes (methanol; Giemsa). Bar = 10 μm.
D. Spleen imprint of circulating macrophage (monocyte). (methanol; Giemsa). Bar = 10 μm.
E. Goblet cells of the buccal cavity (formalin; ABPAS). Bar = 64 μm.
F. Reticular fiber stroma of the liver and hepatopancreas (ethanol; GR). Bar = 57 μm.

1 Erythrocyte (red blood cell)
2 Goblet cell containing sialomucins (blue)
3 Goblet cells containing neutral mucopolysaccharides (red)
4 Granulocyte (neutrophilic)
5 Hepatic portal vein
6 Immature erythrocyte (reticulocyte)
7 Intrahepatic pancreatic acini
8 Lymphocyte (small)
9 Lymphocyte with pseudopods (large)
10 Macrophage (monocyte)
11 Nuclei of the hepatocytes
12 Red blood cells in vein
13 Reticular fibers (black)
14 Thrombocyte, spiked form
15 Thrombocyte with a dumbbell nucleus

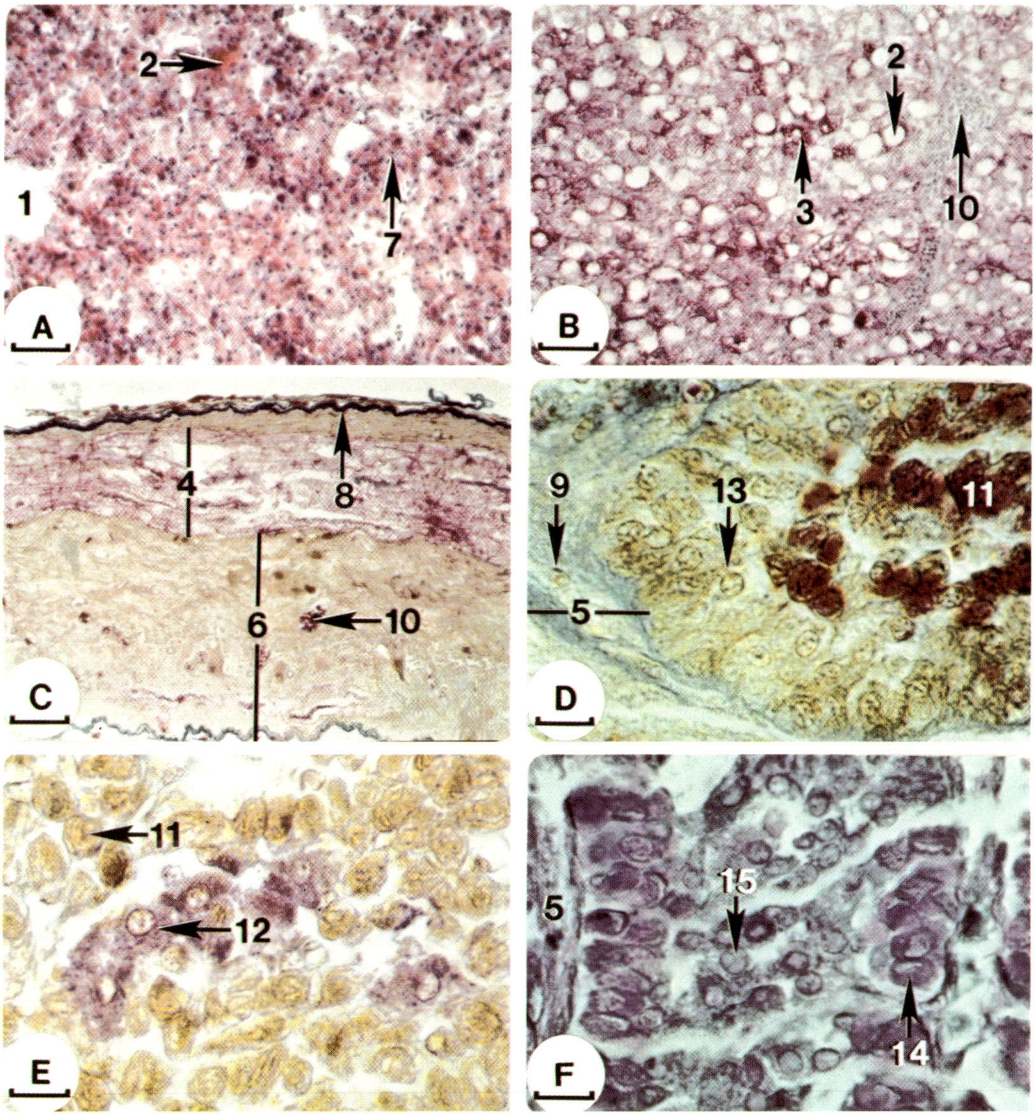

Plate 3. Liver, spinal cord, and pituitary of a 3-year-old striped bass.

A. Accumulated fat vacuoles in the liver parenchyma (formalin; ORO). Bar = 56 μm.
B. Glycogen deposits in the liver parenchyma (ethanol; BC). Bar = 55 μm.
C. Sagittal section of spinal cord (Helly's; Azan). Bar = 58 μm.
D. Rostral pars distalis, female fish (Bouin–Allen's; Azan). Bar = 10 μm.
E. Rostral pars distalis, female fish (Bouin–Allen's; AFH). Bar = 10 μm.
F. Proximal pars distalis, female fish (Helly's; CHP). Bar = 10 μm.

1 Central vein
2 Fat vacuoles (orange-red in **A**)
3 Glycogen granules (red in **B**)
4 Myelinated white matter (red in **C**)
5 Neurohypophysial fibers
6 Nonmyelinated gray matter (yellow in **C**)
7 Nuclei of the hepatocytes
8 Pia arachnoid membrane (leptomeninx)
9 Pituicyte
10 Red blood cells in a vein
11 Type-I cells (prolactin cells)
12 Type-II cells (gonadotrophs)
13 Type-III cells (corticotrophs)
14 Type-IV cells (somatotrophs)
15 Type-V cells (thyrotrophs)

Plate 4. Pituitary, urophysis, and endocrine pancreas of a 3-year-old striped bass.

A. Pars intermedia, female fish (Helly's; CHP). Bar = 10 μm.
B. Pars intermedia, female fish (Helly's; Azan). Bar = 10 μm.
C. Urophysis spinalis (Bouin's; CVOG). Bar = 369 μm.
D. Medullary area of the urophysis spinalis (Bouin's; Azan). Bar = 25 μm.
E. Neurosecretory Dahlgren's cell, in the dorsal urophysis spinalis (Helly's; AFH). Bar = 10 μm.
F. Endocrine pancreatic tissue (Bouin's AFLG). Bar = 20 μm.
G. Endocrine pancreatic tissue (Helly's; PTAH). Bar = 10 μm.

1 Acidophilic colloidal droplets
2 Acinar cells
3 Alpha cells (blue granules in **G**)
4 Beta cells (dark blue cytoplasm in **F**)
5 Connective tissue (leptomeninx)
6 Dahlgren's cell
7 Glial cells
8 Nerve fibers of medulla
9 Neurohypophysial fibers
10 Neurosecretory product
11 Nucleus of Dahlgren's cell
12 Pituicytes
13 Type-II cell (gonadotrophs)
14 Type-VII cell
15 Type-VIII cell (MSH producing cell)
16 Type-IX cell (gonadotrophs)
17 Zymogen granules in acinar cell

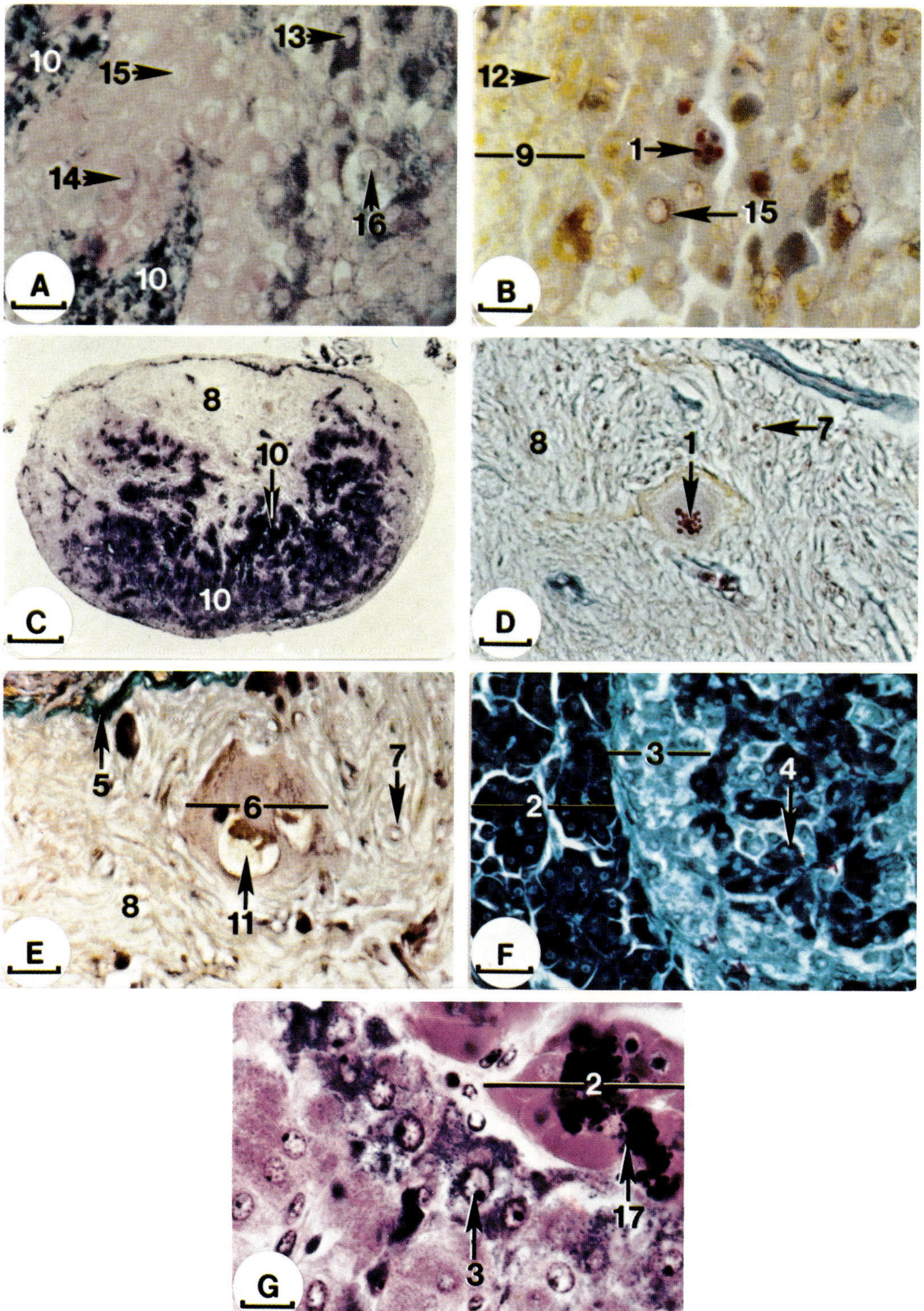

Plate 4

REFERENCES

Agius, C. 1979. The role of melano-macrophage centers in iron storage in normal and diseased fish. Journal of Fish Diseases 2:337–343.

Agius, C. 1980. Phylogenetic development of melano-macrophage centers in fish. Journal of Zoology (London) 191:11–31.

Al-Hussaini, A. H. 1946. The anatomy and histology of the alimentary tract of the bottom-feeder *Mulloides auriflamma* (Forsh). Journal of Morphology 78:121–153.

Al-Hussaini, A. H. 1947. The anatomy and histology of the alimentary tract of the plankton-feeder *Atherina forsali* (Ripp). Journal of Morphology 80:251–286.

Ali, M. A., and M. Anctil. 1976. Retinas of fishes. Springer-Verlag, Berlin, West Germany.

Alperin, I. M. 1966a. Dispersal, migration, and origins of striped bass from Great South Bay, Long Island. New York Fish and Game Journal 13:79–112.

Alperin, I. M. 1966b. Occurrence of yearling striped bass along the south shore of Long Island. New York Fish and Game Journal 13:113–120.

Anderson, B. G., and W. D. Anderson. 1976. Renal vasculature of the trout demonstrated by scanning electron microscopy, compared with canine glomerular vessels. American Journal of Anatomy 145:443–458.

Anderson, B. G., and D. L. Mitchum. 1974. Atlas of trout histology. Wyoming Game and Fish Commission Bulletin 13.

Anderson, D. P. 1974. Diseases of fishes. Book 4: fish immunology. T.F.H. Publications, Neptune, New Jersey, USA.

Ariens Kappers, C. V., G. C. Huber, and E. C. Crosby. 1936–1965. The comparative anatomy of the nervous sytem of vertebrates including man, volumes 1, 2, and 3. Hafner, New York, New York, USA.

Austin, H. M., and O. Custer. 1977. Seasonal migration of striped bass in Long Island Sound. New York Fish and Game Journal 24:53–68.

Bach, R., P. B. Chen, and G. B. Chapman. 1978. Changes in the spleen of the channel catfish *Ictalurus punctatus* Rafinesque induced by infection with *Aeromonas hydrophila.* Journal of Fish Diseases 1:205–217.

Ball, J. N., and B. I. Baker. 1969. The pituitary gland: anatomy and histophysiology. Pages 1–93 *in* W. S. Hoar and D. J. Randall, editors. Fish physiology, volume 2. Academic Press, New York, New York, USA.

Bannister, L. H. 1965. The fine structure of the olfactory surface of teleostean fishes. Quarterly Journal of Microscopical Science 106:333–342.

Barber, L. D., and J. E. M. Westermann. 1975. "Rodlet cells" in *Catostomus commersonnii* (Teleostei: Pisces): secretory cell or parasite? Experimentia 31:924–925.

Barber, L. D., and J. E. M. Westermann. 1978. Occurrence of the periodic acid-Schiff positive granular leucocyte (PAS-GL) in some fishes and its significance. Journal of Fish Biology 12:35–43.

Barber, L. D., J. E. M. Westermann, and D. N. Jensen. 1979. New observations on the rodlet cell (*Rhabdospora thelohani*) in the white sucker *Catostomus commersoni* (Lacépède): LM and EM studies. Journal of Fish Biology 14:277–284.

Barkuloo, J. 1970. Taxonomic status and reproduction of the striped bass (*Morone saxatilis*) in Florida. United States Bureau of Sport Fisheries and Wildlife Technical Paper 44.

Barnett, C. H. 1951. The structure and function of the choroidal gland of teleostean fish. Journal of Anatomy 85:113–119.

Bauer, R. F. 1973. Fine structure of the gill lamellae of euryhaline striped bass *Morone saxatilis.* Journal of the Elisha Mitchell Scientific Society 83(4):207. (Abstract.)

Beatty, D. D. 1975. The role of the pseudobranch and choroid rete mirabile in fish vision. Pages 635–644 *in* M. A. Ali, editor. Vision in fishes. Plenum Press, New York, New York, USA.

Beitch, I. 1962. A histomorphological comparison of the urinary system in serranid fishes *Roccus saxatilis* and *R. americanus.* Master's thesis. University of Richmond, Richmond, Virginia, USA.

Beitch, I. 1963. Striped bass histo-morphological study. Virginia Commission of Game and Inland Fisheries, Federal Aid in Fish Restoration, F-5-R-8 Warmwater Fisheries Management, Job 11, Final Report, Richmond, Virginia, USA.

Belsare, D. K. 1973. Comparative anatomy and histology of the corpuscles of Stannius in teleosts. Zeitschrift fuer Mikroskopisch-Anatomische Forschung (Leipzig) 87:S445–456.

Bently, P. J. 1976. Comparative vertebrate endocrinology. Cambridge University Press, Cambridge, England.

Berlind, A. 1973. Caudal neurosecretory system: a physiologist's view. American Zoologist 13:759–770.

Bern, H., and N. Takasugi. 1962. The caudal neurosecretory system of fishes. General and Comparative Endocrinology 2:96–110.

Bigelow, H., and W. Schroeder. 1953. Fishes of the Gulf of Maine. United States Fish and Wildlife Service Fishery Bulletin 53 (74).

Blake, I. M. 1930. Studies on the comparative histology of the digestive tube of certain teleost fishes. I. A predaceous fish, the sea bass (*Centropristes striatus*). Journal of Morphology and Physiology 50:39–70.

Blake, I. M. 1936. Studies on the comparative histology of the digestive tube of certain teleost fishes. III. A bottom-feeding fish, the sea robin, (*Prionotus carolinus*). Journal of Morphology 60:77–102.

Boddingius, J. 1975. The cell types of the adenohypophysis in the rainbow trout (*Salmo irideus*). A histological study. Holywell Press, Oxford, England.

Bonga, S. E. W., J. A. A. Greven, and M. Veenhuis. 1976. The relationship between the ionic composition of the environment and the secretory activity of the endocrine cell types of Stannius corpuscles in the teleost *Gasterosteus aculeatus*. Cell and Tissue Research 175:297–312.

Bonga, S. E. W., J. A. A. Greven, and N. Veenhuis. 1977. Vascularization, innervation, and ultrastructure of the endocrine cell types of Stannius corpuscles in the teleost *Gasterosteus aculeatus*. Journal of Morphology 153:225–243.

Boynton, W. R., T. T. Polgar, and H. H. Zior. 1981. Importance of juvenile striped bass food habits in the Potomac estuary. Transactions of the American Fisheries Society 110:56–63.

Bradford, A. 1957. The striped bass—Life history and management. Photocopy from Library of W. Whitworth, University of Connecticut, Storrs, Connecticut, USA. (Unpublished manuscript).

Brinn, J. E. 1973. The pancreatic islets of bony fishes. American Zoologist 13:653–655.

Bryant, C. P. 1970. The morphology of the renal systems of the striped bass *Roccus saxatilis* (Walbaum). Anatomical Record 166:284. (Abstract.)

Bryant, C. P., and H. R. Seibel. 1970. Histological and ultrastructural aspects of the pronephric phase of renal development in the larval striped bass *Roccus saxatilis*. Virginia Journal of Science 21:143.

Bryant, C. P., and H. R. Seibel. 1971. Ultrastructural investigation of tubulogenesis in the mesonephros of the striped bass. Anatomical Record 169:285. (Abstract.)

Bucke, D. 1971. Anatomy and histology of the alimentary tract of the carnivorous fish, the pike, *Esox luicius*. Journal of Fish Biology 3:421–431.

Bucke, D. 1972. Some histological techniques applicable to fish tissues. Symposia of the Zoological Society of London 30:153–189.

Burnstock, G. 1959. The innervation of the gut of the brown trout. Quarterly Journal of Microscopical Science 100:199–219.

Burton, D. 1978. Melanophore distribution within the integumentary tissues of two teleost species, *Pseudopleuronectes americannus* and *Gasterosteus aculeatus* form *leiurus*. Canadian Journal of Zoology 56:526–535.

Butler, D. G. 1973. Structure and function of the adrenal gland of fishes. American Zoologist 13:839–879.

Cahn, P. H., editor. 1966. Lateral line detectors. Indiana University Press, Bloomington, Indiana, USA.

Campbell, G., and B. J. Gannon. 1976. The splanchnic nerve supply to the stomach of the trout, *Salmo trutta* and *S. gairdneri*. Comparative Biochemistry and Physiology, C, Comparative Pharmacology 55:51–53.

Catton, W. T. 1951. Blood cell formation in certain teleost fishes. Blood 6:39–60.

Chadwick, H. K. 1962. Annual abundance of young striped bass (*Roccus saxatilis*) in the Sacramento–San Joaquin Delta, California. California Fish and Game 50:69–93.

Chakrabarte, J., R. Scharya, and D. K. Belsare. 1973. Structure of the gall bladder in some freshwater teleosts. Zeitschrift fuer Mikroskopisch-Anatomische Forschung (Leipzig) 87:523–532.

Chao, L. N. 1973. Digestive system and feeding habits of the cunner, *Tautogolabris adspersus*, a stomachless fish. United States National Marine Fisheries Service Fishery Bulletin 71:565–586.

Chapoton, R. B., and J. E. Sykes. 1961. Atlantic coast migration of large striped bass as evidenced by fisheries and tagging. Transactions of the American Fisheries Society 90:13–20.

Cheprakova, Iu. I. 1958. The structure and histogenesis of the pharyngeal teeth in certain fish of the carp species. Doklady Akademii Nauk SSSR Biological Science Section (English translation) 121:630–633.

Chevalier, G. 1978. *In vivo* incorporation of [^{3}H]leucine and [^{3}H]tyrosine by caudal neurosecretory cells of the trout *Salvelinus fontinalis* in relation to osmotic manipulations. A radioautographic study. General and Comparative Endocrinology 36:223–228.

Clark, J. 1968. Seasonal movement of striped bass contingents of Long Island Sound and the New York Bight. Transactions of the American Fisheries Society 97:320–343.

Combs, R. M. 1969. Embryogenesis, histology and organology of the ovary of *Brevoortia patronus*. Gulf Research Reports 2:333–434.

Cooper, J. L. 1952. A histological study of the reproductive organs of crappies (*Pomoxis nigromaculatus* and *Pomoxis annularis*). Transactions of the American Microscopical Society 71:393–404.

Copeland, E. 1951. Function of the glandular pseudobranch in teleosts. American Journal of Physiology 167:775. (Abstract.)

Courtois, L. A. 1976. Hematology of juvenile striped bass, *Morone saxatilis* (Walbaum) acclimated to different environmental conditions. Comparative Biochemistry and Physiology A Comparative Physiology 54:221–223.

Crosby, E., and M. J. Showers. 1969. Comparative anatomy of the preoptic and hypothalamus areas. Pages 61–131 *in* W. Haymaker, E. Anderson, and W. Nauta, editors. The hypothalamus. Charles C. Thomas, Springfield, Illinois, USA.

Curry, E. 1939. The histology of the digestive tubes of the carp (*Cyprinus carpio communis*). Journal of Morphology 65:53–78.

Dalberg, M. D., and D. C. Scott. 1971. Introduction of freshwater fishes in Georgia. Bulletin of the Georgia Academy of Science 29.

Daxboeck, C., and G. F. Holeton. 1978. Oxygen receptors in the rainbow trout, *Salmo gairdneri*. Canadian Journal of Zoology 56:1254–1259.

Dey, W. P. 1981. Mortality and growth of young of the year striped bass in the Hudson River estuary. Transactions of the American Fisheries Society 110:151–157.

Dickson, A. W. 1958. The status of striped bass (*Roccus saxatilis*) (Walbaum) in North Carolina waters. Proceedings of the Annual Conference Southeastern Association of Game and Fish Commissioners 11:264–268.

Dixit, V. P. 1970. Histophysiological studies of the interrenal gland in *Clarias batrachus* Linn. Acta Anatomica 77:310–318.

Dobbin, C. N. 1941. A comparative study of the gross anatomy of the airbladder of ten families of fishes of New York and other eastern states. Journal of Morphology 68:1–29.

Dorfman, D. 1976. Occurrence of a hermaphroditic

white perch (*Morone Americana*). Progressive Fish Culturist 38:45.

Dovel, W. L. 1968. Predation by striped bass as a possible influence on population size of Atlantic croaker. Transations of the American Fisheries Society 97:313–319.

Dovel, W. L., and J. R. Edmonds. 1971. Recent changes in the striped bass (*Morone saxatilis*) spawning sites and commercial fishing areas in upper Chesapeake Bay: possible influencing factors. Chesapeake Science 12:33–39.

Drance, M. C., M. J. Hollenberg, M. Smith, and V. Wylie. 1976. Histological changes in trout testis produced by injections of salmon pituitary gonadotropin. Canadian Journal of Zoology 54:1285–1293.

Dudley, R. G., A. W. Mullis, and J. W. Terrell. 1977. Movements of adult striped bass (*Morone saxatilis*) in the Savannah River, Georgia. Transactions of the American Fisheries Society 106:319–322.

Ellis, A. E., T. S. Hartings, and A. L. S. Munro. 1981. The role of *Aeromonas salmonicida* extracellular products in the pathology of furunculosis. Journal of Fish Diseases 4:41–51.

Engel, D. W., and E. M. Davis. 1964. Relationship between activity and blood composition in certain marine teleosts. Copeia 1964:586–587.

Epple, A. 1967. A staining sequence for A, B, and D cells of pancreatic islets. Stain Technology 42:53–61.

Epple, A., and T. L. Lewis. 1973. Comparative histophysiology of the pancreatic islets. American Zoologist 13:567–590.

Ezeasor, D. N., and W. M. Stokue. 1980. A cytochemical, light and electron microscopic study of the eosinophilic granule cells in the gut of the rainbow trout, *Salmo gairdneri* Richardson. Journal of Fish Biology 17:619–634.

Fänge, R. 1953. The mechanisms of gas transport in the euphosoclist swimbladder. Acta Physiologica Scandinavica 30 (Supplement 110):5–133.

Fänge, R., and D. Grove. 1979. Digestion. Pages 162–241 *in* W S. Hoar, D. J. Randall, and J. R. Brett, editors. Fish physiology, volume 8. Academic Press, New York, New York, USA.

Faulkner, R. C. 1952. A comparative study of the retinae of four serranid fishes, *Lepibema chrysops* (Rafinesque); *Morone interupta* (Gill); *Morone americana* (Gmelin); and *Roccus saxatilis* (Walbaum). Master's thesis. University of Oklahoma, Norman, Oklahoma, USA.

Fearnhead, E. A., and B. C. Fabion. 1971. The ultrastructure of the gill of *Monodactylus argenteus*. Changes in salinity. Oceanographic Research Institute (Durban) Investigational Report 26: 3–39.

Ferguson, H. W. 1976. The relationship between ellipsoids and melano-macrophage centers in the spleen of turbot (*Scophthalmus maximus*). Journal of Comparative Pathology 86:377–380.

Fink, W. L. 1981. Ontogeny and phylogeny of tooth attachment modes in actinopterygian fishes. Journal of Morphology 167:167–184.

Fiore, M. S. H., R. E. Mancini, and E. D. P. Roberts. 1973. New atlas of histology. Lea and Febiger, Philadelphia, Pennsylvania, USA.

Flock, A. 1967. Ultrastructure and function in the lateral line organs. Pages 163–198 *in* P. H. Cahn, editor. Lateral line detectors. Indiana University, Bloomington, Indiana, USA.

Flood, M. T., R. F. Nigrelli, and J. F. Gennaro, Jr. 1975. Some aspects of the ultrastructure of the stäbchendrüsenzellen, a peculiar cell associated with the endothelium of the bulbus arteriosus and with other fish tissues. Journal of Fish Biology 7:129–138.

Forester, C. R., A. E. Peden, and R. M. Wilson. 1972. First record of the striped bass (*Morone saxatilis*) in British Colombia waters. Journal of Fisheries Research Board of Canada 29:337–339.

Gabe, M. 1976. Histological techniques. Masson, Springer-Verlag, Berlin, West Germany.

Gona, O. 1979. Mucous glycoproteins of teleostean fish: a comparative histochemical study. Histochemistry 11:709–718.

Goodson, L. F. 1964. Diet of striped bass at Millerton Lake, California. California Fish and Game 50:307.

Greene, C. W. 1912. Anatomy and histology of the alimentary tract of the king salmon. United States Bureau of Fisheries, Bulletin 32:73–100.

Grier, H. J. 1981. Cellular organization of the testis and spermatogenesis in fishes. American Zoologist 21:345–357.

Grizzle, J. M., and W. A. Rogers. 1976. Anatomy and histology of the channel catfish. Auburn University Agricultural Experiment Station, Auburn, Alabama, USA.

Grünberg, V. W., and G. Hager. 1978. Zur Ultrastruktur der Stäbchendrüsenzellen (rodlet cells, pear-shaped cells) im Bulbus anteriosus der Karpfen, *Cyprinus carpio* L. (Pisces: Cyprinidae). Anatomische Anzeiger 143:227–290.

Hafeez, M. 1971. Light microscopic studies on the pineal organ in teleost fishes with special regard to its function. Journal of Morphology 134:281–314.

Hale, P. A. 1965. The morphology and histology of the digestive system of two freshwater teleosts, *Poecilia reticulata* and *Gasterosteus aculeatus*. Journal of Zoology (London) 146:132–149.

Hall, F. G. 1924. The functions of the swimbladder of fishes. Biological Bulletin (Woods Hole) 47:79–126.

Ham, A. W. 1974. Histology, 7th edition. J. B. Lippincott, Philadelphia, Pennsylvania, USA.

Harder, W. 1975. Anatomy of fishes. E. Schweizerbart'sche Verlagsbuchhandlung (Nägele v. Obermiller), Stuttgart, West Germany.

Hatten, S. R. 1942. Striped bass spawning areas in California. California Fish and Game 28:65.

Hentschel, H. 1978. The kidney of the Prussian carp, *Carassius auratus gibelio* (Cyprinidae). III. Glycogen-rich cells in the distal segment of nephronic tubule. Tissue and Cell 10:319–330.

Heubach, W., R. J. Toth, and A. M. McCready. 1963. Food of young of the year striped bass (*Roccus saxatilis*) in the Sacramento-San Joaquin River system. California Fish and Game 49:224–239.

Hinton, D. E., R. L. Snipes, and M. W. Kendall. 1972. Morphology and enzyme histochemistry in the liver of largemouth bass *Micropterus salmoides*. Journal of the Fisheries Research Board of Canada 29:531–534.

Hoar, W. S. 1965. Comparative physiology: hormones and reproduction in fishes. Annual Review of Physiology 27:51–70.

Hoar, W. S., and D. J. Randall, editors. 1969. Fish physiology, volume 2. Academic Press, New York, New York, USA.

Hoar, W. S., and D. J. Randall, editors. 1971. Fish physiology, volume 5. Academic Press, New York, New York, USA.

Hogue, J. J., R. Wallus, and L. K. Kay. 1977. Natural reproduction by striped bass in Kentucky and Barkey Reservoirs. Journal of the Tennessee Academy of Science 52:77–79.

Hollis, E. H. 1952. Variations in the feeding habits of the striped bass, *Roccus saxatilis* (Walbaum), in Chesapeake Bay. Bulletin of the Bingham Oceanographic Collection, Yale University 14:111–131.

Honma, Y., S. Shioda, and S. Yoshie. 1977. Changes in the thyroid gland associated with the diadromous migration of the threespine stickleback. Japanese Journal of Ichthyology 24:17–25.

Howe, D., and J. Gutknecht. 1978. Role of urinary bladder in osmoregulation in marine teleost, *Opsanus tau*. American Journal of Physiology 235:R48–R54.

Hughes, G. M., and A. V. Grimstone. 1965. The fine structure of the secondary lamellae of the gills of *Gadus pollachius*. Quarterly Journal of Microscopical Science 106:343–353.

Hughes, J. S. 1975. Striped bass, *Morone saxatilis* (Walbaum), culture investigations in Louisiana with notes on sensitivity of fry and fingerlings to various chemicals. Louisiana Fish and Wildlife Commission Bulletin 13, New Orleans, Louisiana, USA.

Humason, G. 1972. Animal tissue techniques. W. H. Freeman, New York, New York, USA.

Hunter, C. R., and P. L. Nayudu. 1978. Surface folds in superficial epidermal cells of three species of teleost fish. Journal of Fish Biology 12:163–166.

Hurley, D. A., and K. Fisher. 1966. The structure and development of the external membrane in young eggs of the brook trout, *Salvelinus fontinalis*. Canadian Journal of Zoology 44:173–190.

Iwai, T. 1967. Structure and development of lateral line cupulae in teleost larvae. Pages 27–44 *in* P. H. Cahn, editor. Lateral line detectors. Indiana University Press, Bloomington, Indiana, USA.

Jaiswol, A. G., and D. K. Belsare. 1973. Comparative anatomy and histology of the caudal neurosecretory system in teleosts. Zeitschrift fuer Mikroskopisch-Anatomische Forschung (Leipzig) 87:589–609.

James, M. F. 1946. Changes in bluegill and bass gonads, *Lepomis macrochirus* and *Huro salmoides*. Journal of Morphology 79:63–91.

Jansen$_1$, W. F., R. A. deWeger, R. A. Woutersen, H. van Loveren, and J. C. van de Kamer. 1976. The saccus dorsalis of the rainbow trout, *Salmo gairdneri*: Richardson. Histological, cytochemical, electron microscopical, and autoradiographical observations. Cell and Tissue Research 167:467–491.

Jansen$_2$, W. F., H. van Loveren, R. A. Woutersen, and R. A deWeger. 1976. Enzyme-cytochemistry of the saccus dorsalis of the rainbow trout, *Salmo gairdneri*: Richardson. Histochemistry 48:293–306.

Johnson, D. E., J. L. Torrence, R. P. Elde, G. E. Baver, B. D. Noe, and D. J. Fletcher. 1976. Immunohistochemical localization of somatostatin, insulin, and glucogen in the principle islets of the angler-fish (*Lophius americanus*) and the channel catfish (*Ictalurus punctata*). American Journal of Anatomy 147:119–124.

Johnson, R. K., and T. S. Y. Koo. 1975. Production and distribution of striped bass (*Morone saxatilis*) eggs in the Chesapeake and Delaware canal. Chesapeake Science 10:39–55.

Johnson, W. C., and A. J. Calhoun. 1952. Food habits of California striped bass. California Fish and Game 38:531–534.

Jose, T. M., and A. G. Sathyanesan. 1977. Hypothalamus-hypophysial neurosecretory and vascular system of the teleost *Labeo rohita* (Ham). Anatomischer Anzeiger 142:424–434.

Junqueira, L., M. H. Alves Lima, and E. C. Farias. 1978. Carotenoid and pterin pigment localization in fish chromatophores. Stain Technology 53:91–94.

Kendall, M. W., and W. E. Hawkins. 1975. Hepatic morphology and acid phosphatase localization in the channel catfish. Journal of the Fisheries Research Board of Canada 32:1459–1464.

Kendall, M. W., and D. E. Hinton. 1974. Renal tubular morphology in the channel catfish (*Ictalurus punctatus*) kidney. Journal of the Fisheries Research Board of Canada 31:346–347.

Kernehan, R. J., M. R. Headrick, and R. E. Smith. 1981. Early life history of striped bass in the Chesapeake and Delaware Canal and vicinity. Transactions of the American Fisheries Society 110:137–150.

Khalilov, F. 1966. Some material on the histology and histochemistry of the pancreas and liver of teleost fish. Problems in Ichthyology (Journal of Ichthyology, English translation of Voprosy Ikhtiologii) 8:240–249.

Khanna, S. S., and H. R. Singh. 1967. Histology and histochemistry of the saccus vasculosus in some teleosts (Pisces). Acta Anatomica 67:304–311.

Kikucki, S. 1977. Mitochondria-rich (chloride) cells in the gill epithelia from four species of stenohaline freshwater teleosts. Cell and Tissue Research 180:87–98.

Kirschner, L. B. 1977. The sodium chloride secreting cells in marine vertebrates. Pages 427–452 *in* B. L. Gunta, R. B. Moreton, J. L. Oschmal, and B. J. Wall, editors. Transport of ions in water and animals. Academic Press, New York, New York, USA.

Kleerekoper, H. 1969. Olfaction in fishes. Indiana University, Bloomington Indiana, USA.

Klein, C. 1977. Ultrastructural and cytochemical bases for the identification of cell types in the endocrine pancreas of teleosts. Pages 289–346 *in* National review of cytology. Academic Press, New York, New York, USA.

Koo, T. 1970. Striped bass fishery in the Atlantic States. Chesapeake Science 11:73–93.

Koo, T. S. Y., and D. E. Ritchie. 1973. Growth of juvenile striped bass (*Morone saxatalis*) as determined by tagging and recapture. Sport Fishery Abstracts 19:169.

Koo, T. S. Y., and J. S. Wilson. 1972. Sonic tracking striped bass in the Chesapeake and Delaware Canal.

Transactions of the American Fisheries Society 101:453–462.

Kreutzburg, G. W., and G. W. Gross. 1977. General morphology and axonal ultrastructure of the olfactory nerve of the pike, *Esox lucius*. Cell and Tissue Research 181:443–457.

Kristal, J. 1946. The exocrine pancreatic tissue of seven teleosts. South African Journal of Medical Sciences 11:79–87.

Laerm, J. 1976. The development, function, and design of amphicoelous vertebrae in teleost fishes. Zoological Journal of the Linnean Society 58:237–254.

Lagler, K. F., J. E. Bardach, R. R. Miller, and D. R. M. Passino. 1977. Ichthyology, 2nd edition. John Wiley and Sons, New York, New York, USA.

Laurent, P., and S. Dunel. 1976. Functional organization of the teleost gill. I. Blood pathways. Acta Zoologica (Stockholm) 57:189–204.

Laurent, P., and S. Dunel. 1978. Histophysiologie—relations anatomiques des ionocytes (cellules à chlorure) avec le compartiment veineux branchial: définition de deux types d'épithélium de la branchie des poissons. Comptes rendus Academic de Sciences Paris, Série D:1447–1450.

Leake, L. 1975. Comparative histology. Academic Press, New York, New York, USA.

Leeson, T. S., and C. R. Leeson. 1970. Histology, 2nd edition. W. B. Saunders, Philadelphia, Pennsylvania, USA.

Leonard, J. B., and R. G. Summers. 1976. The ultrastructure of the integument of the American eel, *Anguilla rostrata*. Cell and Tissue Research 171:1–30.

Lester, R. J. G., and B. A. Daniels. 1976. The eosinophilic cell of the white sucker, *Catostomus commersoni*. Journal of the Fisheries Research Board of Canada 33:139–144.

Levene, C., and P. Feng. 1964. Critical staining of pancreatic alpha granules with phosphotungstic acid hematoxylin. Stain Technology 34:39–44.

Lewis, R. M. 1957. Comparative study of populations of striped bass. United States Fish and Wildlife Service Special Scientific Report Fisheries 204.

Lowenstein, O. 1971. The larbyrinth. Pages 207–240 *in* W. S. Hoar and D. J. Randall, editors. Fish physiology, volume 5. Academic Press, New York, New York, USA.

Luna, L. G., editor. 1967. Manual of histologic staining methods of the Armed Forces Institute of Pathology, 3rd edition. McGraw-Hill, New York, New York, USA.

Lund, W. A., Jr. 1957. Morphometric study of the striped bass (*Roccus saxatilis*). United States Fish and Wildlife Service Special Scientific Report Fisheries 216.

Lyall, A. H. 1957. Cone arrangement in teleost retinae. Quarterly Journal of Microscopical Science 98:189–201.

Mahajan, C. L., and J. M. S. Dheer. 1980. An autoradiographic and cytochemical study of erythropoiesis in a fresh water fish *Channa punctatus* Block. Journal of Fish Biology 17:641–648.

Manooch, C. S. 1973. Food habits of yearling and adult striped bass, *Morone saxatilis*, from Albemarle Sound, North Carolina. Chesapeake Science 14:73–86.

Mansueti, R. 1958. The development of anal spines and soft-rays in young striped bass, *Roccus saxatilis*. Chesapeake Biological Laboratory Contribution 113, Maryland Department of Research and Education, Annapolis, Maryland, USA.

Mansueti, R. J. 1961. Age, growth, and movement of the striped bass, *Roccus saxatilis*, taken in size selective fishery gear in Maryland. Chesapeake Science 2:9–36.

Markle, D. F., and G. C. Grant. 1970. The summer food habits of young striped bass in three Virginia rivers. Chesapeake Science 11:50–54.

Marshall, A. J., and B. Lofts. 1956. The Leydig-cell homologue in certain teleost fishes. Nature (London) 177:704–705.

Massmann, W. H., and A. L. Pacheco. 1961. Movements of striped bass tagged in Virginia waters of Chesapeake Bay. Chesapeake Science 2:37–44.

Mattey, D. L., R. Moate, and M. Morgan. 1978. Comparison of "pseudobranch" type and "chloride" type cells in the pseudobranch of marine, freshwater, and euryhaline teleosts. Journal of Fish Biology 13:535–542.

Mattey, D. L., M. Morgan, and D. E. Wright. 1979. Distribution and development of rodlet cells in the gills and pseudobranch of the bass *Dicentrachus labray* (L). Journal of Fish Biology 15:363–370.

Mayberry, L. F., A. A. Marchiondo, J. E. Ubelaker, and D. Kazia. 1979. *Rhadospores thelohani* Languesse 1895 (Apiromplexa): new host and geographic records with taxonomic considerations. Journal of Protozoology 26:168–178.

McLaren, J. B., J. C. Cooper, T. B. Hoff, and V. Lander. 1981. Movements of Hudson River striped bass. Transactions of the American Fisheries Society 110:158–167.

McLean, J. R., and S. Nilsson. 1981. A histochemical study of the gas gland innervation in the Atlantic cod, *Gadus morhua*. Acta Zoologica 62:187–194.

McMillan, P. J., W. M. Hooker, B. A. Roos, and L. J. Deftos. 1976. Ultimobranchial gland of the trout (*Salmo gairdneri*). I. Immunohistology and radioimmunoassay of calcitonin. General and Comparative Endocrinology 28:313–319.

McNulty, J. A. 1976. A comparative study of the pineal complex of the deepsea fish *Bathylagus wesethi* and *Nezumia liolepis*. Cell and Tissue Research 172:205–225.

McNulty, J. A., and B. G. Nafpaktitis. 1977. Morphology of the pineal complex in seven species of lantern fishes (Pisces: Myctophidae). American Journal of Anatomy 150:509–530.

Meader, R. G. 1939. The forebrain of bony fishes. Proceedings of the Koninklijke Nederlandse Akademie van Wetenschappen 42:657–670.

Merriman, D. 1940. The osteology of the striped bass (*Roccus saxatilis*). Annals and Magazine of Natural History, Series 11:55–64.

Merriman, D. 1941. Studies on the striped bass (*Roccus saxatilis*) of the Atlantic coast. United States Fish and Wildlife Service Fishery Bulletin 50:1–77.

Moore, C. J., and D. T. Burton. 1974. Movement of striped bass (*Morone saxatilis*) tagged during late fall

50(35).

in Chesapeake Bay, Maryland. Sport Fishery Abstracts 19:286.

Moore, C. J., and D. T. Burton. 1975. Movements of striped bass (*Morone saxatilis*) tagged in Maryland waters of Chesapeake Bay. Transactions of the American Fisheries Society 104:703–709.

Morgan, R. P., T. S. Y. Koo, and G. E. Krantz. 1973. Electrophoretic determination of population of the striped bass (*Morone saxatilis*) in the upper Chesapeake Bay. Transactions of the Amerian Fisheries Society 102:21–32.

Morrison, C. M., and P. H. Odense. 1978. Distribution and morphology of the rodlet cell in fish. Journal of the Fisheries Research Board of Canada 35:101–116.

Moser, G. H. 1967. Seasonal histological changes in the gonads of *Sebastodes paucispinis* Ayers, an ovoviviparous teleost (Family Scorpaenidae). Journal of Morphology 123:329–354.

Nagahama, Y., H. A. Bern, B. A. Doneen, and R. S. Nishioka. 1975. Cellular differentiation in the urinary bladder of the euryhaline marine fish, *Gillichthys mirabilis*, in response to environmental salinity changes. Development, Growth and Differentiation 17:367–381.

Nandi, J. 1962. The structure of the interrenal gland in teleost fishes. University of California Publications in Zoology 65:129–212.

Nichols, P. 1966. The striped bass. United States Fish and Wildlife Service Bureau of Commercial Fisheries Fishery Leaflet 592.

Nichols, P. R., and R. V. Miller. 1967. Seasonal movement of striped bass, *Roccus saxatilis* (Walbaum), tagged and released in the Potomac River, Maryland 1959–1961. Chesapeake Science 8:102–124.

Nieuwenhuys, R. 1962. Trends in the evolution of the actinopterygian forebrain. Journal of Morphology 111:69–88.

Nieuwenhuys, R. 1963. Comparative anatomy of the actinopterygian forebrain. Journal für Hirnforschung 6:171–192.

Nieuwenhuys, R. 1967. Comparative anatomy of the cerebellum. Progress in Brain Research 25:1–94.

Oguri, M. 1976. Histochemical observations on the dark brown pigment granules found in the kidney tissue of rainbow trout. Bulletin of the Japanese Society of Scientific Fisheries 42:1223–1227.

Oguri, M., and H. Sokabe. 1968. Juxtaglomerular cells in the teleost kidneys. Bulletin of the Japanese Society of Scientific Fisheries 34:882–888.

Olivereau, M., and J. Olivereau. 1977. Effects of transfer to sea water and back to fresh water on the histological structure of the eel kidney. Journal of Comparative Physiology 115:223–239.

Olivereau, M., and J. Olivereau. 1978. Prolactin, hypercalcemia, and corpuscles of Stannius in seawater eels. Cell and Tissue Research 186:81–96.

Orsi, J. J. 1971. The 1965–1967 migration of the Sacramento–San Joaquin estuary striped bass population. California Fish and Game 57:257–267.

Otto, R. S. 1975. Isoenzyme systems of the striped bass (*Morone saxatilis*) and congeneric percichthyid fishes. Doctoral dissertation. University of Maine, Orono, Maine, USA.

Ottosen, P. D. 1978. Ultrastructure and segmentation of microdissected kidney tubules in the marine flounder, *Pleuronectes platessa.* Cell and Tissue Research 190:27–45.

Pang, P. K. T. 1971. Calcinonin and ultimobranchial glands in fishes. Journal of Experimental Zoology 178:89–100.

Parry, G., and F. G. T. Holliday. 1960. An experimental analysis of the function of the pseudobranches in teleost. Journal of Experimental Biology 37:344–354.

Patt, D. I., and G. R. Patt. 1969. Comparative vertebrate histology. Harper and Row, New York, New York, USA.

Pearson, J. C. 1938. The life history of the striped bass, or rockfish, *Roccus saxatilis* (Walbaum). United States Bureau of Fisheries Bulletin 28(49):825–851.

Pearson, R., and L. Pearson. 1976. The vertebrate brain. Academic Press, London, England.

Perks, A. M. 1969. The neurohypophysis. Pages 112–205 *in* W. S. Hoar and D. J. Randall, editors. Fish physiology, volume 2. Academic Press, New York, New York, USA.

Popper, A. N. 1977. A scanning electron microscopic study of the sacculus and lagena in the ears of fifteen species of teleost fishes. Journal of Morphology 153:397–418.

Pouwells, E. 1976. On the development of the cerebellum of the trout, *Salmo gairdneri.* Doctoral dissertation. Catholic University, Nijmegen, Denmark.

Radovich, J. 1963. Effect of ocean temperature on the seaward movement of striped bass, *Roccus saxatilis*, on the Pacific Coast. California Fish and Game 49:191–206.

Radtke, L. D., and J. L.Turner. 1967. High concentration of total dissolved solids block spawning migration of striped bass, *Roccus saxatilis*, in the San Joaquin River, California. Transactions of the American Fisheries Society 96:405–407.

Raney, E. 1952. The life history of the striped bass. Bulletin of the Bingham Oceanographic Collection, Yale University 14(1):5–97.

Raney, E. C., and D. P. DeSylva. 1953. Racial investigations of the striped bass (*Roccus saxatilis* [Walbaum]). Journal of Wildlife Management 17:495–509.

Raney, E. C., and W. S. Wolcott. 1955. Races of the striped bass "*Roccus saxatilis*" (Walbaum) in southeastern U.S. Journal of Wildlife Management 19:44–450.

Rathjen, W. F., and L. C. Muller. 1957. Aspects of the early life history of the striped bass (*Roccus saxatilis*) in the Hudson River. New York Fish and Game Journal 4:43–60.

Reifel, W. C., and A. A. Travill. 1977. Structure and carbohydrate histochemistry of the esophagus in ten teleostean species. Journal of Morphology 152:303–314.

Reno, H. W. 1966. The infraorbital canal, its lateral-line ossicles and neuromasts in the minnows *Notropis volucellus* and *N. buchanan.* Copeia 1966:403–413.

Reyer, H. U. 1977. The role of the swim-bladder in vertical movement of fishes (*Carassius auratus, Salmo gairdneri,* and *Tilapia mariae*). Biology of Behavior 2:109–128.

Ritchie, D. E., and T. S. Y. Koo. 1973. Movement of juvenile striped bass in the estuary as determined by tagging and recapture. Sport Fishery Abstracts 19:173.

Roberts, R. J. 1975. Melanin-containing cells of teleost fish and their relation to disease. Pages 399–428 *in* W. E. Ribelin and G. Migaki, editors. The pathology of fishes. University of Wisconsin Press, Madison, Wisconsin, USA.

Roberts, R. J., editor. 1978. Fish pathology. Bailliere Tindall, London, England.

Robinson, J. B. 1960. The age and growth of striped bass, *Roccus saxatilis*. California Fish and Game 46:279–290.

Rogick, M. D. 1931. Studies on the comparative histology of the digestive tube of certain teleost fishes. Journal of Morphology and Physiology 52:1–23.

Ronsivalli, L. 1976. The role of fish in meeting the world's food needs. Marine Fisheries Review 40(1):18–20.

Ross, L. G. 1979. The haemodynamics of gas resorption from the physoclist swimbladder: the structure and morphometrics of the oval in *Pollachius virens* (L.). Journal of Fish Biology 14:261–266.

Sage, M. 1973. The evolution of thyroidal function in fishes. American Zoologist 13:899–905.

Satchell, G. H. 1971. Circulation of fishes. Cambridge University Press, London, England.

Schaefer, R. H. 1968. Size, age, composition and migration of striped bass from the surf waters of Long Island. New York Fish and Game Journal 15:1–51.

Schaefer, R. H. 1970. Feeding habits of striped bass from the surf waters of Long Island. New York Fish and Game Journal 17:1–17.

Schnitzlein, H. M. 1962. The habenula and the dorsal thalamus of some teleosts. Journal of Comparative Neurology 118:225–267.

Schnitzlein, H. M. 1977. The telencephala of division I of the teleost fishes. Journal für Hirnforsch 18:157–178.

Schreck, C. B., and P. F. Scanlon. 1977. Endocrinology in fisheries and wildlife biology and management. Fisheries (Bethesda) 2(3):20–27.

Schreibman, M. P., J. F. Leatherland, and B. A. McKeown. 1973. Functional morphology of the teleost pituitary gland. American Zoologist 13:719–742.

Schwerdtfeger, W. K., and J. Bereiter-Hahn. 1978. Transcient occurrence of chloride cells in the abdominal epidermis of the guppy *Poecilia reticulata* Peters, adapted to sea water. Cell and Tissue Research 191:463–471.

Scott, H. R. 1952. Rapid staining of beta cell granules in pancreatic islets. Stain Technology 27:267–268.

Scruggs, G. D. 1957. Reproduction of resident striped bass in Santee-Cooper Reservoir, South Carolina. Transactions of the American Fisheries Society 85:144–159.

Scruggs, G. D., and J. C. Fuller. 1955. Indications of a freshwater population of striped bass, *Roccus saxatilis* (Walbaum), in Santee-Cooper Reservoir. Proceedings of the Annual Conference Southeastern Association of Game and Fish Commissioners 8:64–69.

Shapovalov, L. 1936. Food of striped bass. California Fish and Game 22:261–271.

Sis, R. F., P. J. Ives, D. M. Jones, D. H. Lewis, and W. E. Haensly. 1979. The microscopic anatomy of the oesophagus, stomach, and intestine of the channel catfish, *Ictalurus punctatus*. Journal of Fish Biology 14:179–186.

Smith, F. M., and D. R. Jones. 1978. Localization of receptors causing hypoxic bradycardia in trout (*Salmo gairdneri*). Canadian Journal of Zoology 56:1260–1265.

Smith, H. M. 1907. Fishes of North Carolina. North Carolina Annual Economic Survey 2:271.

Stevens, R. E. 1958. The striped bass of the Santee-Cooper Reservoir. Proceedings of the Annual Conference Southeastern Association of Game and Fish Commissioners 11:253–264.

Storch, V. N., and U. N. Welsch. 1970. Electron microscopic observations on the taste-buds of some bony fishes. Archivum Histologicum Japonicum 32:145–153.

Suckling, J. A. 1967. Trunk lateral line nerves: some anatomical aspects. Pages 45–52 *in* P. H. Cahn, editor. Lateral line detectors. Indiana University Press, Bloomington, Indiana, USA.

Tamura, E., and Y. Honma. 1977. Histological changes in the organs and tissues of the gobiid fishes throughout their life-span. VIII. Seasonal changes in the thymus of four species of gobies. Bulletin of the Japanese Society of Scientific Fisheries 43:963–974.

Tavolga, W. M. 1976. Sound reception in fishes. Dowden, Hutchinson and Ross, Stroudsburg, Pennsylvania, USA.

Tesoriero, J. V. 1977. Formation of the chorium (zona pellucida) in the teleost. *Oryzias latipes*. I. Morphology of early oogenesis. Journal of Ultrastructural Research 59:282–291.

Thomas, J. L. 1907. The diet of juvenile and adult striped bass, *Roccus saxatilis*, in the Sacramento-San Joaquin River system. California Fish and Game 53:44–62

Thurmond, T. 1979. Histology and pathology of the alimentary tract of the American eel (*Anguilla rostrata*). Master's thesis. University of Connecticut, Storrs, Connecticut USA.

Tokumaru, M., and A. Ferri. 1970. Histochemistry of the pigments found in the liver, spleen, and kidney of fresh-water fish. Revista Brazileira de Biologia 30:163–171.

Trent, W. L., and W. W. Hassler. 1966. Feeding behavior of adult striped bass in relation to stages of sexual maturity. Chesapeake Science 7:189–192.

Tresselt, E. F. 1952. Spawning grounds of striped bass or rock, *Roccus saxatilis* (Walbaum), in Virginia. Bulletin of the Bingham Oceanographic Collection, Yale University 14(1):98–110.

Turner, J. L. 1976. Striped bass spawning in the Sacramento and San Joaquin Rivers in central California from 1962–1972. California Fish and Game 62:106–118.

Turner, J. L., and H. K. Chadwick. 1972. Distribution and abundance of young of the year striped bass, *Morone saxatilis*, in relation to river flow in the Sacramento-San Joaquin estuary. Transactions of the American Fisheries Society 101:442–452.

United Nations Food and Agriculture Organization.

1975. Yearbook of fishery statistics, volume 40. United Nations Food and Agriculture Organization, Rome, Italy.

United States Department of Commerce. 1972–1973. Fishery statistics. Unites States National Marine Fisheries Service Statistical Digest 66.

Unsicker, K., T. Polonius, R. Lindmar, K. Löffelholz, and U. Wolf. 1977. Catecholamines and 5-hydroxytryptamine in corpuscles of Stannius of the salmonid, *Salmo irideus*. II. A study correlating electron microscopical, histochemical and chemical findings. General and Comparative Endocrinology 31:121–132.

Vladykov, V. D., and D. H. Wallace. 1938. Is the striped bass (*Roccus lineatus*) of Chesapeake Bay a migrating fish? Transactions of the American Fisheries Society 67:67–86.

Vladykov, V. D., and D. H. Wallace. 1952. Studies of the striped bass, *Roccus saxatilis* (Walbaum), with special reference to the Chesapeake Bay region during 1936–38. Bulletin of the Bingham Oceanographic Collection, Yale University 14(1):132–177.

Walker, E. R., S. F. Fidler, and D. E. Hinton. 1981. Morphology of the buccopharyngeal portion of the gill in the fathead minnow, *Pimephales promelas*. The Anatomical Record 200:67–81.

Walker, T J. 1967. History, histological methods, and details of the structure of the lateral line of the walleye surfperch. Pages 13–25 *in* P. H. Cahn, editors. Lateral line detectors. Indiana University Press, Bloomington, Indiana, USA.

Wallace, R. A., and K. Selman. 1981. Cellular and dynamic aspects of oocyte growth in teleosts. American Zoologist 21:325–343.

Wassersug, R. J., and R. K. Johnson. 1976. A remarkable pyloric caecum in the evermannellid genus *Coccorella* with notes on gut, structure and function in alepisauroid fishes. Journal of Zoology (London) 179:273–289.

Weber, D. D., and M. H. Schiewe. 1976. Morphology and function of the lateral line of juvenile steelhead trout in relation to gas-bubble disease. Journal of Fish Biology 9:217–233.

Weinreb, E. L., and N. M. Bilstad. 1955. Histology of the digestive tract and adjacent structures of the rainbow trout, *Salmo gairdneri irideus*. Copeia 1955:194–204.

Weiss, R. E., and N. Watabe. 1978. Studies on the biology of fish bone. II. Bone matrix changes during resorption. Comparative Biochemistry and Physiology A, Comparative Physiology 61:245–251.

Welsch, U., and V. Storch. 1976. Comparative animal cytology and histology. Sidgwick and Jackson, London, England.

Westin, D. T. 1978. Serum and blood from adult striped bass, *Morone saxatilis*, Estuaries 1:123–125.

Westin, D. T., and B. A. Rogers. 1978. Synopsis of biological data on the striped bass *Morone saxatilis* (Walbaum) 1792. University of Rhode Island, Marine Technical Report 67, Kingston, Rhode Island, USA.

Westman, J. R., and D. H. Wallace. 1954. Migrating pattern and racial structure of Atlantic Coast striped bass. Transactions of the North American Wildlife Conference 19:376–398.

Whitear, M. 1977. A functional comparison between the epidermis of fish and of amphibians. Symposia of the Zoological Society of London 39:291–313.

Whitear, M., A. K. Mittal, and E. B. Lane. 1980. Endothelial layers of fish skin. Journal of Fish Biology 17:43–65.

Wirtanen, L. T., and R. H. Ray. 1971. Striped bass, *Morone saxatilis* (Walbaum), 1970 report on the development of essential requirements for production. United States Fish and Wildlife Service, Atlanta, Georgia, USA.

Wittenberg, J. B., D. E. Copeland, R. L. Haedrick, and J. S. Child. 1980. the swimbladder of deep-sea fish: the swimbladder wall is a lipid-rich barrier to oxygen diffusion. Journal of the Marine Biological Association of the United Kingdom 60:263–276.

Wong, W. C., and C. K. Tan. 1981. Fine structure of the myenteric and submucous plexuses in the stomach of a coral fish, *Chelman rostratus* Cuvier. Journal of Anatomy 126:291–301.

Woodhead, A. D. 1977. Aging changes in the liver of two poecilid fishes, the gupp *Poecilia* (*Lebistes*) *reticulata* and the Amazon molly *P. formasa*. Experimental Gerontology 13:37–45.

Woodhull, C. 1947. Spawning habits of striped bass (*Roccus saxatilis*) in California waters. California Fish and Game 33:97–102.

Woolcott, W. S. 1957. Comparative osteology of serranid fishes of the genus *Roccus*. Copeia 1957:1–11.

Yamamoto, M., and K. Ueda. 1977. Comparative morphology of fish olfactory epithelium. I. Salmoniformes. Bulletin of the Japanese Society of Scientific Fisheries 43:1163–1174.

Yamamoto, M., and K. Ueda. 1978a. Comparative morphology of fish olfactory epithelium. II. Clupeiformes. Bulletin of the Japanese Society of Scientific Fisheries 44:855–859.

Yamamoto, M., and K. Ueda. 1978b. Comparative morphology of fish olfactory epithelium. III. Cypriniformes. Bulletin of the Japanese Society of Scientific Fisheries 44:1201–1206.

Yamamoto, M., and K. Ueda. 1978c. Comparative morphology of fish olfactory epithelium. IV. Anguilliformes and Myctophiformes. Bulletin of the Japanese Society of Scientific Fisheries 44:1207–1212.

Yamamoto, M., and K. Ueda. 1978d. Comparative morphology of fish olfactory epithelium. V. Gasterosteiformes, Channiformes, Synbranchiformes. Bulletin of the Japanese Society of Scientific Fisheries 44:1309–1314.

Yamamoto, M., and K. Ueda. 1978e. Comparative morphology of fish olfactory epithelium. VI. Siluriformes. Zoological Magazine (Tokyo) 87:254–261.

Yamamoto, M., and K. Ueda, 1978f. Comparative morphology of fish olfactory epithelium. VII. Gadiformes, Lophiformes, and Gobiesociformes. Journal of the Faculty of Science University of Tokyo Section IV Zoology 14:115–125.

Yamane, S., and J. Yamada. 1977. Histological changes of the ultimobranchial gland through the life history of the Masu salmon (*Oncorhynchus masou*). Bulletin of the Japanese Society of Scientific Fisheries 43:375–386.

Yoakim, E. G., and J. M. Grizzle. 1980. Histological,

histochemical, and ultrastructural studies on the interrenal and chromafin cells of the fathead minnow *Pimephales promelus* Rafinesque. Journal of Fish Biology 17:477–494.

Yoffey, J. M. 1929. A contribution to the study of the comparative histology and physiology of the spleen, with reference chiefly to its cellular constituents. I. In fishes. Journal of Anatomy 63:314–344.

Youson, J. H. 1976. Fine structure of granulated cells in the posterior cardinal and renal veins of *Amia calva* L. Canadian Journal of Zoology 54:843–851.

Youson, J. H., and D. C. Butler. 1976. Fine structure of the adrenocortical homolog and the corpuscles of Stannius of *Amia calva* L. Acta Zoologica (Stockholm) 57:217–230.

Youson, J. H., D. C. Butler, and. A. T. C. Chan. 1976. Identification and distribution of the adrenocortical homolog, chromaffin tissue, and corpuscles of Stannius in *Amia calva* L. General and Comparative Endocrinology 29:198–211.

Zaccone, G. 1977. Histology, innervation, and histochemistry of the ultimobranchial gland in the Mexican cave fish *Anoptichthys jordani* Hubbs et Innes (Teleostei Characidae). Acta Histochemica 58:31–38.

Zieske, E., R., Melinkat, H. Breucher, and J. Kux. 1976. Ultrastructural studies on the epithelia of the olfactory organ of cyprinodonts (Teleostei, Cyprinodontoidea). Cell and Tissue Research 172:245–267.

Zotterman, Y. 1967. The neural mechanism of taste. Progress in Brain Research 23:135–154.

Zottoli, S. J. 1978. Comparative morphology of the Mauthner cell in fish and amphibians. Pages 13–45 *in* D. Faber and H. Horn, editors. Neurobiology of the Mauthner cell. Raven Press, New York, New York, USA.

Zyznar, E. 1975. Tapeta lucida and the organization of visual cells in teleosts. Pages 299-304 *in* M. A. Ali, editor. Vision in fishes. Plenum Press, New York, New York, USA.

Subject Index for Figures and Plates